Nursing Education
in Thanatology:
A Curriculum Continuum

ABOUT THE EDITORS

Florence E. Selder, PhD, RN, is Associate Professor and Urban Research Center Scientist, University of Wisconsin at Milwaukee. She is in private psychotherapy practice at the Midwest Center for Human Services, Milwaukee. Dr. Selder, co-editor of *Human and Ethical Issues in the Surgical Care of Patients With Life Threatening Diseases*, has contributed many articles on thanatology and nursing to professional journals.

Virginia W. Barrett, DPH, MEd, RN, is a research scientist for Columbia University Center for Geriatrics and Gerontology. Dr. Barrett is involved in numerous research projects concerned with memory impaired elderly.

Marilyn M. Rawnsley, DNSc, RN, is Professor in the Department of Nursing Education at Teacher's College, Columbia University, New York, New York. She serves as a consultant to General Hospital in New York/New Jersey in the areas of nursing research and psychosocial aspects of oncology patient care.

Austin H. Kutscher, PhD, is President of The Foundation of Thanatology, and Professor of Dentistry (in Psychiatry) at the College of Physicians and Surgeons, Columbia University, in New York City. His clinical and teaching activities have focused on psychosocial aspects of life-threatening illness and bereavement; cancer diagnosis, therapy, and management; and pharmacotherapeutics. Dr. Kutscher is the editor of *Loss, Grief, & Care*.

Carole A. Lambert, MPA, RN, is Director of Admissions at Marymount Manhattan College in New York, New York. Ms. Lambert is also a member of Columbia University Seminar.

Marcia Fishman, MA, RN, maintains a part-time practice in New York City, counseling patients, their families, and caregivers on issues related to living with dying, death, and bereavement. She has taught, lectured, and published on various topics in thanatology.

Mary Kachoyeanos, EdD, RN, is Associate Professor in the School of Nursing at the University of Wisconsin in Milwaukee. She has researched the responses of parents and siblings to sudden versus anticipated death of a child. Dr. Kachoyeanos is also a research consultant to Children's Hospital in Milwaukee, Wisconsin.

Nursing Education in Thanatology: A Curriculum Continuum

Florence E. Selder, Virginia W. Barrett,
Marilyn M. Rawnsley, Austin H. Kutscher,
Carole A. Lambert, Marcia Fishman,
and Mary Kachoyeanos
Editors

Jill C. Crabtree
Editor for the Foundation of Thanatology

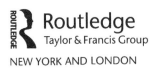
Routledge
Taylor & Francis Group

NEW YORK AND LONDON

First published 1990 by
The Haworth Press, Inc. 10 Alice Street, Binghamton, NY 13904-1580

This edition Published 2014 by Routledge
711 Third Avenue, New York, NY 10017, USA
2 Park Square, Milton Park, Abingdon, Oxfordshire OX14 4RN

First issued in paperback 2015

Routledge is an imprint of the Taylor & Francis Group, an informa business

Nursing Education in Thanatology: A Curriculum Continuum has also been published as *Loss, Grief & Care*, Volume 4, Numbers 1/2 1990.

Library of Congress Cataloging-in-Publication Data

Nursing education in thanatology : a curriculum continuum / Florence E. Selder ... [et al.], editors.
    p. cm.
    "Has also been published as Loss, grief & care, volume 4, numbers 1/2, 1990" – T.p. verso.
    Inlcudes bibliographical references.
    ISBN 0-86656-996-0 (alk. paper)
    1. Nursing. 2. Terminal care. 3. Nursing – Psychological aspects. 4. Death – Psychological aspects. 5. Thanatology. I. Selder, Florence.
    [DLM: 1. Attitude to Death – nurses' instruction. 2. Curriculum. 3. Education, Nursing. 4. Terminal Care – nurses' instruction. 5. Thanatology – nurses' instruction. W1 LO853F v. 4 no. 1/2 / WY 18 N9737]
RT87.T45N88 1990
610.73'61 – dc20
DNLM/DLC
for Library of Congress
               90-4470
               CIP

ISBN 13: 978-1-138-88185-3 (pbk)
ISBN 13: 978-0-86656-996-5 (hbk)

Nursing Education in Thanatology: A Curriculum Continuum

CONTENTS

ABOUT THE CONTRIBUTORS

Rinda Alexander, PhD, Associate Professor, BNS Program, Department of Nursing, Purdue University-Calumet, Hammond, IN.

Pat Underwood Babcock, RN,EdD, Acting Chairperson and Associate Professor, Department of Nursing, Purdue University-North Central, Westville, IN.

Virginia W. Barrett, RN, PhD, Community Health Nursing Consultant, Columbia University, New York State Office of Mental Health, New York, NY.

Sister Mary Ann Borello, MA, Professor of Sociology, Suffolk County Community College, Brentwood, NY.

Lucy G. Bruce, MEd, Associate Professor, Division of Interdisciplinary Studies, School of Allied Health Sciences, The University of Texas Medical Branch, Galveston, TX.

John G. Bruhn, PhD, Dean and Professor, Preventive Medicine and Community Health, School of Allied Health Sciences, The University of Texas Medical Branch, Galveston, TX.

Mary A. Crosley, RN, MS, Coordinator of Nursing Program, Suffolk County Community College, Brentwood, NY.

Catherine O. D'Amico, RN, MA, Former Director, School of Practical Nursing for Staff Development, The Weiler Hospital of the Albert Einstein College of Medicine, Division of Montfiore Medical Center, Bronx, NY.

Lisa Danto, RN, Public Health Nurse, Washtenaw County Department of Human Services, Public Health Division, Ann Arbor, MI.

Margaret R. Edwards, RN, MSN, Assistant Professor of Nursing, College of Health Professions, Wichita State University, Wichita, KS.

Marcia Fishman, RN, MPH, Formerly, Nursing Practice Advocate, The Presbyterian Hospital in the City of New York, NY; Private Practice and Counseling, New York, NY.

Evelyn R. Hayes, RN, PhD, Chairperson, Department of Nursing Science, College of Nursing, University of Delaware, Newark, DE.

Mary Kachoyeanos, RN, PhD, Associate Professor, School of Nursing, University of Wisconsin, Milwaukee, WI.

Austin H. Kutscher, President, The Foundation of Thanatology, New York, NY; Professor of Dentistry (in Psychiatry), Department of Psychiatry, College of Physicians and Surgeons, Columbia University, New York, NY.

Carole A. Lambert, RN, MPA, Formerly, Psychiatric Nurse Clinician, Jewish Home and Hospital for the Aged, Bronx, New York; Director of Admissions, Marymount Manhattan College, New York, NY.

Madeline E. Lambrecht, RN, MSN, Assistant Professor, Department of Nursing Science, College of Nursing, University of Delaware, Newark, DE.

D. Lisa Leonard, PhD, Associate Dean for Curricula Affairs; Associate Professor, Division of Interdisciplinary Studies, School of Allied Health Sciences, The University of Texas Medical Branch, Galveston, TX.

Mary Dee McEvoy, RN, PhD, Robert Wood Johnson Clinical Nurse Scholar, University of Pennsylvania School of Nursing, Philadelphia, PA.

Mostafa H. Nagi, PhD, Professor of Sociology, Bowling Green State University, Bowling Green, OH; Visiting Professor, Kuwait University College of Arts.

Roberta M. Orne, RN, MS, Assistant Professor, University of Connecticut, Storrs, CT.

Marilyn M. Rawnsley, RN, DNSc, Visiting Professor, Department of Nursing Education, Teachers College, Columbia University, New York, NY.

Mary A. Seidel, RN, MA, Doctoral Student, Department of Sociology, University of Washington, Seattle, WA; Coordinator of Staff Development, Children's Hospital Medical Center, Seattle, WA.

Florence E. Selder, RN, PhD, Associate Professor and Urban Research Center Scientist, University of Wisconsin; Clinical Associate, Midwest Center for Human Sciences, Milwaukee, WI.

Note

This compilation originated from a symposium sponsored by the Foundation of Thanatology, titled, "The Thanatology Curriculum for Schools of Medicine, Nursing, and Allied Health Professions (Content of, Educational Approaches to, Introduction of and or Augmentation of)," held at Columbia-Presbyterian Medical Center, New York, NY in March of 1985.

Nursing Education in Thanatology: A Curriculum Continuum

SECTION I:
TEACHING ASPECTS AND THE THANATOLOGY CURRICULUM CONTENT

Considerations in Teaching Thanatology

Florence E. Selder

The formal teaching of thanatology in schools for health care professionals is generally overlooked and ill-defined. It is assumed to be taught when "it" happens. The "it" may be the first time a student is confronted with the death of a patient. A deliberate, purposeful inclusion of thanatology in the curriculum will insure prepared health care professionals are ready to assist patients and/or their families during an emotionally difficult time. Utilizing a specific approach, a context of language and intervention strategies will facilitate the effective teaching of thanatology. Furthermore, an awareness of caregiver behaviors and factors of student supervision will strengthen the teaching program.

Considerations of what and when (content) and how and where (process) to teach thanatology, are functions of the approach. The content, or didactic material, may be fixed exclusively in a course on death and dying. It may be integrated into related courses such as an ethics course, a course on terminal diseases, intensive care or

1

E.R. nursing, or a discussion of disabilities. It may also be informally interwoven throughout the curriculum according to spontaneous student interest or need.

Process, or the context in which the information is transmitted and learning acknowledged, can include a lecture presentation, an experiential program, or a combination of both. Decisions as to which orientation to employ will be influenced by parameters such as class and room size, time available for both content and experience, the availability of experimental resource materials, and the student's familiarity and practice with aspects of thanatology.

The very minimum information for any one curriculum should include a description of at least one theory of individual response to loss, the impact on family members and the caregiver, and one's particular professional role and responsibility relating to the physiological process of dying, care of the patient, and, impact on survivors. The minimum provision of context or process should be an opportunity for students to respond to the didactic information presented.

If, in the curriculum, only lecture is allocated to thanatological study, the recommended approach for the novice or inexperienced student is to provide many process experiences. Beginning students have an absence of clinical experience and will be less able to comprehend and utilize the content in a meaningful way. The use of a film or participatory exercise compensates for this experiential deficiency. Most students do have personal experiences with loss in their individual histories and relationships. Through process activities, these experiences can be drawn upon in reflection and inquiry for greater understanding of thanatology.

In contrast, students who have had clinical experience may best be served with the presentation of a specific conceptual framework (e.g., stages of dying) within which to integrate their experiences.

An effective approach that meets a variety of students' background and knowledge, is to integrate content and process in a three-credit course. One credit may be allocated to required attendance at lectures and films during a weekend seminar. The remaining two credits may be allocated to participation in various small group activities such as writing farewell letters or epitaphs, making videotaped messages for loved ones, creating clay or art products, or dramatizing the experience of being dead.

Placing the content in a conceptual framework of language is vital to the student's ability to organize the many facts or notions about loss, death and dying. Providing a language for students furnishes them with a map to understand the complexity of thanatology. The particular framework chosen is less important than the fact that one needs to be selected. Whatever the selected framework, students will share a common base of knowledge through which they will be able to communicate their experiences. The framework can be further utilized for assessment interventions.

A number of conceptual frameworks exist. The stages of dying framework is one example of a language context and includes Kübler-Ross's (1969) stages of dying. Further, life transition theory (Selder, in press) is useful to examine persons' responses to loss. Each of these models provides a means to understand and verbalize experiences in response to loss. An eclectic approach which encompasses multiple frameworks can be utilized with increased experience and understanding.

Appropriate intervention strategies stem from and are determined by the selected conceptual framework. To illustrate, examples are presented here relating to the life transition theory concepts of of strategies Reactivation and Missed Options. Reactivation is the awareness of thoughts, feelings and sensations reminiscent of those that occurred earlier. For instance, a woman may hear noises upstairs and momentarily conclude her husband is getting up. Immediately, she realizes her husband is dead and has been dead for the past few weeks. When the phenomenon of reactivation occurs it is disconcerting to the individual; the woman feels as she did when she first discovered her husband had died. In addition to the distress of reliving the loss, people view reactivation as a sign that they have not made any progress with their grieving.

Appropriate interventions in this example are to describe the phenomenon of reactivation as a common response to loss. In addition, indicating that it is a repeated experience that decreases in intensity with subsequent episodes, provides comfort and assurance to the patient.

Another intervention illustrated from life transition theory to missed options. Missed options are those behaviors in which a person previously claimed competency. For instance, a missed option for a person with a spinal cord injury is the option of walking again. The point at which a person realizes a missed option varies from individual to individual. Arriving at the realization is a process in itself that causes much uncertainty, fear and distress.

Appropriate interventions in this instance are to assist the person in identifying unavailable options. In addition, helping the person discover a means to minimize the intrusiveness of the missed option will reduce the fear and uncertainty.

Caregiver behaviors have a significant influence on intervention strategies and health care professionals' beliefs about loss. Wright's (1960) concepts of spread effect and requirement for mourning demonstrate this point. The spread effect results when any deviation of person's behavior and personality is seen as being more than just one deviation. For instance a student may assume that because a blind person cannot see, he also cannot hear, though there is no connection. Similarly, we speak very loudly to older clients, assuming that they have lost hearing along with aging. Requirement for mourning implies that whomever we consider unfortunate is suffering. Assumptions that a person has can have a spread effect on patient care. Thus, a student may assume that all patients who are dying will always feel devastated. Hence, they will not allow for the possibility that the patient may have found some meaning in his or her dying and is not devastated. In addition, a patient's care will be influenced by a student who assumes that a dying person is hard of hearing or doesn't hear at all, who is unable to laugh, tell jokes, have cognitive functioning or feel empathy for others.

It is necessary to emphasize that the caregiver has the responsibility to care for himself/herself. In working with persons who are dying, bereaved, or who are dealing with loss, it is likely that one may become depleted or overwhelmed. There are many strategies to support oneself and these may be discussed in the curriculum. Essentially, it is the responsibility of caregivers to care for themselves so that their care of others is not depleting.

Supervision is the final consideration in teaching thanatology concepts. Supervision in a clinical setting is self-evident and in existence. Supervision is less evident in a classroom setting. Supervision guarantees that a means is established to ensure that students' responses are known by the teacher. Subsequent guidance may be provided if appropriate. Reaction papers are one-page self-reports on course content, films, exercises and guest speakers. Reaction papers will indicate to the faculty the status of students' experiences, concerns and responses. For instance, a student in one reaction paper did indicate that she goes to the cemetery to talk to her mom and she wonders if this is normal behavior. Students can be reassured in the faculty's written response to their reaction paper about their concerns. If numerous students have these concerns, then the comments can be used as a basis for class discussion.

In summary, there are several practical considerations to be addressed when deciding to include thanatology concepts in a curriculum. Including a determined approach, language, and interventions will maximize teaching efforts. Awareness of caregiver behaviors and student supervision will further ensure successful teaching of thanatology in the health care curriculum.

REFERENCES

Kübler-Ross, E. (1969). *On death and dying*. New York: Macmillan Co.
Selder, F. (In press). Women and loss: Dealing with uncertainty. In Tallmer, M. et al. (Eds.). *Implications of death and loss for women*. New York: Foundation of Thanatology.
Wright, B. (1960). *Physical disability – a psychological approach*. New York: Harper & Row.

Concepts of Thanatology in the Nursing Curriculum

Rinda Alexander

In the past two decades much attention has been focused on the concepts and dynamics of thanatology. The burgeoning literature in the study of death and dying has, however, tended to focus on the narrow view. As a consequence the large view of the human condition tends to be fractured (Jackson, 1979). At the same time, significant advances have been achieved in the area of medical diagnoses and treatment of the terminally ill. What is unfortunate, however, is that emotional support for the individuals and the survivors (including health care providers) has not kept pace with the technical and medical advances made in treating the terminally ill.

The dying process and the state of death affect both the social and psychological roles of the dying individual. Nonetheless, it is significant that when the individual health professional comes into contact with the dying client, considerable insecurity still exists as to how to appropriately deal with the social and psychological needs of both dying clients and their significant others. Therefore, an understanding of the concepts of thanatology is essential to the terminally ill, their significant others, and holistic health care providers. This is particularly salient for the nurses who provide long term care and have intensive contact with the dying person. Through providing the student nurse with such concepts, better holistic care can be given throughout their careers.

Death education should be very much concerned with the process of living as well as the process of dying. Thanatology in the nursing curriculum can therefore motivate health care providers to take the holistic view of death and dying not only for the client, but also for themselves. Most importantly, educated nurses can then focus on

7

the quality of life for themselves and for others in a less stereo-typical manner (McGrory, 1978).

Nurses react to death personally before they react professionally. Attitudes toward death are culturally learned, and in the American culture there is the tendency to deny death. Other personal reactions have their basis in the psychological maturity and personality characteristics of the individual nurse. Care given the client is influenced by this personal reaction. The nurse, along with the physician, serves as the gatekeeper for many clients during the dying process, and, in the role of gatekeeper, the nurse can help the client achieve a peaceful death. However, whether or not the nurse can help the dying client achieve a peaceful death largely depends on the nurse's orientation toward this role and how he or she has personally experienced death and the dying process.

The therapeutic use of the self is not necessarily in conflict with therapeutic use of technology (Feifel 1959). The holistic nursing professional combines care addressed to the disease process with care addressed to the person. It is important that the terminally ill be provided an opportunity to continue their positive self-growth as long as they live. Death education within the nursing curriculum can therefore be a strong stimulus to accept the terminally ill as being alive until they are actually dead. It is imperative that nurses as primary health care providers avoid an "already dead" approach to both clients and their significant others. The process of death education can prepare the health care provider to be better prepared to assume the technical and emotional advocacy role for the terminally ill and their survivors.

It is important to note that nurses in every clinical setting will inevitably encounter the dying process. Even nurses working in health maintenance areas care for the chronically ill, the dying and the recently bereaved survivors.

Learning to help dying clients and their families demands personal involvement of the health care professional. The professional health care provider who has been educated about the concepts of thanatology and effective living as well as dying, can provide consistent and compassionate care for both the dying individual and his or her significant others. This process will enable the dying individual to complete the process of dying with less trauma to both him/herself and others (Alexander 1979).

In recent years a trend toward multidisciplinary education has emerged (McGrory 1978). With the increase of such educational offerings, the value and contributions of each profession can be used more readily. This facilitates physiological, psychological and social support for the terminally ill.

In teaching concepts of thanatology, whether within a discipline or in a multidisciplinary setting, faculty must anticipate students' difficulties and provide individual counseling for the professional student when and where appropriate. When "studying" the death process, students can go through the same emotions as the dying individual. These intense emotional reactions can be extremely difficult for the student to acknowledge and to handle in a therapeutic manner that facilitates the student's own positive self-growth. This is especially true if the student is already depressed, is having family difficulties, or has a dying family member. It is important that the death educator be adept at counseling and crisis intervention. At the same time, death educators will be more effective at their task if, indeed, they have dealt with their personal feelings, fears, and negative attitudes toward dying.

It has been reported in the literature that some students do have times during the death education process when they need to seek additional counseling. Leviton (1975) cites three major reasons that students seeking such counseling: (1) concern over impending or past death of a loved one; (2) suicidal thinking; and (3) thanatophobia, or preoccupation with fears of personal death.

It is evident from two different semesters of death education I conducted, that students who were prone to depression did, indeed, become depressed or more depressed during the presentation of intense death education concepts. Also, students seeking individual counseling during the semester were representative of the three categories noted by Leviton (Alexander 1979).

Benton (1978) addressed this same issue and stated that many of the students in his classes had personal and/or professional experience with death which had resulted in unresolved feelings of grief that came to the forefront during the death education courses.

Individual death educators cannot provide all the answers nor can they make promises of a "hereafter"; what they can do, however, is to help students understand the concepts and dynamics of thanatology which can, in turn, help the health care provider recognize the psychological, social, and cultural aspects of an "appropriate death."

It is important to recognize that those who care for the dying also need to mourn the loss of clients and to work through the grief process. Considerable effort should be made to help individual students recognize their own needs. Also, students should be presented with therapeutic means of coping with the stress of working with the dying and their families. Nurse educators can help nursing professionals overcome barriers to the grief process and its resolution by including more grief work in the nursing school curricula. Through such a process students can get in touch with their own feelings about death—their own and that of others (Alexander 1979).

Stage theories of death have been contributed to the field of thanatology by such theorists as Kübler-Ross (1969) and Lindemann (1972). Although such theories have been useful in stimulating scholarly work and experimental processes in death education, it is important to realize that not all individuals go through each stage in approaching death. Nonetheless, these theories do provide professionals with the means of understanding individual reactions of the terminally ill, significant others and health care professionals. A framework is thereby identified wherein therapeutic interventions can occur.

The education process can help individual health professionals to recognize their own limitations. The nurse is expected to give physical care, understanding, and emotional support. There are limiting factors such as immense emotional strains that must be recognized. Furthermore, there are no standard answers that can be given to many of the questions asked by clients, by families, and even by the nurse.

Nurses cannot avoid death. As nurse professionals examine their own attitudes toward death and dying they can be more therapeutic with others who are experiencing the process of death and dying.

Teaching death education is different from presenting most other courses. The process of emotional growth can often be identified in the class and can become an especially gratifying experience for students and faculty. The feedback from learning becomes immediate and is a positive influence for further growth.

It is expected that nurses who have taken a course on death will interact with the dying patient and the family in a more confident and therapeutic manner. Nurses who have been involved with the death education process and have not yet personally experienced death should find the occurrence of death less emotionally threatening when they first encounter death professionally. In turn, the client, the family, and society will be the benefactors of such a process. If a more honest pattern of dealing with death can be achieved, emotional suffering should be less debilitating and recovery from grief more readily achieved by all the individuals involved. Death education has been demonstrated to be effective in achieving such goals. The effective death educator does indeed contribute to improving the quality of life for society generally, and facilitates the "appropriate death" desired by most clients, survivors and, indeed, the professional nurses who also desire a peaceful death for themselves.

REFERENCES

Alexander, R. (1979). "Death education: Need and approach." Unpublished manuscript.

Benton, R. (1978). *Death and Dying and Practice in Patient Care.* New York: D. Van Nostrand Company.

Feifel, H. (1959). *The Meaning of Death.* New York: McGraw-Hill.

Jackson, E. (1979). "Bereavement and grief." In H. Wass (Ed.), *Dying: Facing the Facts.* New York: McGraw-Hill.

Kübler-Ross, H. (1969). *On Death and Dying.* New York: Macmillan Company.

Leviton, D. (1975). "Education for death or death becomes less a stranger." *OMEGA, 6* (3), 183-191.

Lindemann, E. (1972). "Symptomotology and management of acute grief." *American Journal of Psychiatry, 8,* 101-148.

McGrory, A. (1978). *A Well Model Approach to Care of the Dying Client.* New York: McGraw-Hill.

University of Michigan's School of Nursing Curriculum Related to Issues of Death and Dying

Lisa Ann Danto

The Bachelor of Science in Nursing (BSN) curriculum at the University of Michigan is based on the conceptual framework of adaptation linking the four concepts of person, health, environment, and nursing together. Science-oriented courses are taught primarily during the first two years of the program, and clinical courses, categorized by groups of clientele, are scheduled during the third and fourth years, with nursing theory and courses from the liberal arts integrated throughout the entire four-year program.

During the first year, students take a course entitled Life Span Development. This course reviews content related to growth and development throughout the life span. An emphasis on "object attachment" and "object loss" provides the theory related to death and dying. Kübler-Ross and other theorists are used to describe the grief process and its application throughout the life span. For example, the loss of home and the loss of mobility would be considered common phenomena for the aging, and would be identified as issues related to loss and grief. The focus is not on death and dying, but is more concerned with loss and the person's response to loss, be it situational or developmental. This theory serves as a foundation for the nursing curriculum, and an attempt is made to integrate it throughout the rest of the nursing program, as it is applied to the clinical setting (Erickson 1985).

It is not until the second year, during Basic Concepts of Nursing I and II, that students are first introduced to the clinical setting. These clinical hours ("in-clinical") are very limited and all take place at the University of Michigan Main Hospital. Some of the clinical hours include a seminar and a lab. In addition, students spend clinical hours at various community placements ("out-clinicals") with the elderly population and with children to identify developmental stages, learn rapport with clients, and practice and develop skills related to trust, self-esteem, empathy, love and belonging, safety and security, etc. At this time, students are learning the "nursing process" and the concept of "teaching and learning," with an emphasis on assessment and basic nursing skills. The stress and anxiety of the study is at its highest at this stage of the nursing program. This is directly related to having a heavy course load combined with an unfamiliar clinical setting requiring many new and different skills.

I was fortunate to be in the first student group at the sophomore level allowed to begin our first in-clinical experience on the oncology/hematology unit. There were eight of us in the group out of a class of approximately 100 students. This was *not* my first experience with the dying, but it was perhaps my first *professional* experience. Looking back, I think my primary concern as a nursing student was more for my own performance and survival than for the needs of the dying. This is not to say that I overlooked the dying process, but I feel that I was not developmentally prepared to conceptualize this experience as a nursing student.

During the entire sophomore year, two-and-a-half hours of lecture time and four hours of seminar time are devoted to issues of death and dying. Approximately one-and-a-half of these two-and-a-half lecture hours are reserved for a special speaker who has devoted her professional nursing practice to hospice care. She shares some of her experiences and the needs she has identified for these clients and their families. Students are usually touched by the compassion and personalized care she has for people who are experiencing loss and grief. The seminar time is directed toward students' own personal attitudes, experiences, and emotions related to death and dying, loss, and grief. These seminars vary in content because they are conducted by different clinical instructors or by members of the faculty. There are generally five to ten students in a group. Also, there is a chapter entitled "Nursing the Person with Loss" which is included in the present course textbook, *Introduction to Person-Centered Nursing* (Lindberg et al. 1983).

It is hoped that students will learn how to talk to people and how to gather their own information, including how to be supportive, how to identify the needs of the family, how to identify the needs of the clients experiencing a life crisis (such as loss and grief), and how to assess all of these needs (Hunter 1985).

The junior and senior year is presently on a nine-week rotating clinical schedule. The junior year clinical rotations are Nursing Care of the Child-Bearing Family ("Obstetrics"), Nursing Care of the Child-Rearing Family ("Pediatrics"), and Mental Health Nursing ("Psych"). Students take these in different sequences based on a lottery system, and they are located at various institutions. Coinciding with each of these rotations is a series of "core" courses. The purpose of these core courses is to reinforce concepts that are common to nursing regardless of the setting. The core courses in the junior year are Adaptation of the Family ("Family"), Methods and Measurements in Nursing Settings ("Research"), and Group Concepts ("Groups").

The senior year consists of Nursing Care of the Adult ("Med/ Surg"), Family and Community Health Nursing ("Community Health"), and Nursing Management ("Management") clinical rotations. The core courses in the senior year are Synthesis of the Nursing Process ("Synthesis"), Health Problems of Contemporary Society ("Epidemiology"), Social, Political & Professional Issues ("Nursing Issues"), and Leadership and Decision Making ("Leadership"). In all the junior and senior year nursing courses, the content related to death and dying is limited.

In particular, the Obstetrics course discusses the high risk infant, premature infancy, and infants born with anomalies. There is content related to the loss and grief felt by parents who give birth to a "nonperfect" child. A lecture on ethical issues is provided. However, topics vary from year to year. Some have included such topics as keeping infants on respirators, infertility and the sense of loss and grief at being unable to bear a child, and the parent's response to a stillborn child (Judd 1985). Depending on the circumstances, issues of death and dying may be discussed during the clinical experience as the occasion arises.

In the Pediatric course, there is no specific lecture related to death and dying, except for discussion of medical problems which may alter a family's well-being, such as juvenile arthritis, or may cause an early unexpected death, such as Sudden Infant Death Syndrome (Grishaw 1985). Clinical seminars provide a list of topics from which students may choose to research, write, and present a paper. Each group consists of eight to ten students.

This was my first formal introduction to thanatology because I chose to do research on the topic of "children's concepts of death." I did a survey of the literature concerning children's concepts of death and related these to Erikson's theory of growth and development from infancy to adolescence. We were limited to ten pages or less (a monumental task); therefore, I briefly described each developmental stage according to Erikson, and included nursing interventions useful for dealing with children and their families at each developmental level. Another student chose the topic of "adolescents' response to terminal illness." It is important to note that these topics are randomly chosen by individual students from each seminar; therefore, the seminar content varies among students.

The Mental Health course and the Family core course do not directly address issues of death and dying (Friedl 1985); however, they do refer to individual and family crisis intervention and problem-solving techniques. During the Mental Health clinical seminar or during clinical experience, discussion of death and dying may occur, but that depends on the clients or the occasion. The other junior year core courses, Research and Groups, do not necessarily include issues of death and dying, except as mentioned as an example or as part of a case study.

As for the senior year, little content is included on death and dying. The Medical/Surgical nursing curriculum is based on Orem's theory of "self care" and focuses more on the acute and rehabilitative care of the ill. There is content concerning chronic illness, but not necessarily terminal illness. The following personal experience will help to illustrate how unprepared a number of us were, even at the senior level, to deal with the issue of death and dying.

During my clinical rotation, I was taking care of a woman who was dying (she was designated as a "no code"). My first response to the situation was, "So what am I supposed to do?" I felt helpless and lost in terms of what type of nursing interventions were appropriate for someone of her status. Because of a problem with communication with my instructor, I received very little guidance and support. In addition, I was also responsible for another patient who had multiple needs; therefore, I was unable to spend as much time as I would have liked with the woman who was dying, but did spend enough time to have become very attached to her (as most of the staff had). When she finally died (when I was still responsible for her nursing care), it was interesting to see how everyone responded.

My needs at this time were to have a moment to say "good-bye" to this woman and possibly to perform her postmortem care. I felt relieved for her because she had finally found an end to her suffering. Instead of having the opportunity to vent how I really felt, I was angry because my instructor reminded me that I had another patient to take care of. My instructor was very insensitive to what my needs and priorities were. I felt robbed of my values and powerless to do anything at the time. I practically had to "sneak" into the room so I could say good-bye to her myself, and for a moment I was able to observe the staff nurse doing the postmortem care.

The staff nurse who was ultimately responsible for this woman's nursing care had hoped that the patient wouldn't die on her shift (an unfortunate inconvenience for her!). The students around me were extremely supportive and shared my feelings of loss and frustration, except for one student who had also taken care of her in the past. This particular student could not understand why the woman had been designated as "no code" to begin with and firmly believed all along that this woman was going to get better. For this student it was a particularly difficult situation to comprehend. I think that this is primarily related to this student's upbringing and immaturity. However, it is also reflective of the lack of opportunity for students to experience and learn issues related to death and dying and loss and grief in the nursing school's curriculum.

The Community Health clinical course does not include content related to death and dying issues, unless there is application for case study based on the clients at the student clinical placement (Mars 1985). The Management clinical course does not examine issues of death and dying at all. As for the senior core courses (described below), there is the possibility that issues of death and dying may be discussed, but it is not inherent in the curriculum.

In Synthesis, students learn how to develop their own theory and research based on three to four professional nurse/client relationships. During my course, some topics included discussions of stress, loss, grief, power, control, etc., but they varied in depth and length. Epidemiology focuses on health problems of contemporary society and students research and write a paper and present a topic of their choice using the "prevention model" as a format. Topics related to death and dying in my course were only indirectly related to either disease processes or mortality statistics. In Nursing Issues, there is content related to ethical decision making which *may* discuss issues of death and dying in the form of case studies which are only used as examples. The Leadership course does not address anything at all related to death and dying.

This survey of the University of Michigan's Bachelor of Science in Nursing program has sought to identify what is or is not provided to prepare students for issues surrounding death and dying. The design of the program encourages students to explore outside the curriculum and apply the knowledge that they have gained during the program to several settings. The curriculum's limitation is that it does not allow students enough opportunities to explore these issues and to discuss them at length.

I believe that creativity is needed if any changes are to occur in the curriculum related to issues of death and dying. A graduate level course on Thanatology could be a vital step, provided that direct and open communication with the undergraduate program takes place. Investing in or developing a personalized computer program dealing with issues of death and dying, such as has been explored by other nursing schools, may be useful for students trying to learn about these issues. Educating the faculty regarding issues of death and dying, and how to approach students who are facing clinical situation, is essential.

Issues of death and dying surround us almost every day of our lives; yet they affect us differently depending on a variety of factors. Awareness of these issues should be constant, especially with the growing number of persons diagnosed with a terminal illness. The first step in the right direction would be to educate the administrators of the nursing school regarding the definition of "thanatology," since five of the six department coordinators did not know the meaning of the word when I contacted them about this subject!

REFERENCES

Erickson, H. (March-May 1985). Personal communication.
Friedl, M. (March, 1985). Personal communication.
Grishaw, C. (February-March, 1985). Personal communication.
Hunter, M. (March, 1985). Personal communication.
Judd, J. (March, 1985). Personal communication.
Lindberg, J. B., Hunter, M. L., & Kruszewski, A. Z. (1983). *Introduction to Person-Centered Nursing*. Philadelphia: J. B. Lippincott Company.
Mars, S. (March, 1985). Personal communication.

Cremation in the Thanatology Curriculum

Margaret R. Edwards

Cremation is growing in acceptability and use in most Western nations. Indeed, in the United States the percentage of people who choose to be cremated has increased dramatically during the past 15 years. This change has been attributed primarily to issues of economics, aesthetics, and convenience. Nevertheless, there is a lack of understanding of cremation and its various implications, both among the lay public and among health care providers.

This article is not a testimonial promoting cremation. All of us must make our own personal decisions in this regard. It is our obligation as health care educators, however, to provide a curriculum that prepares students in the health professions to support the client who is confronted with this decision. If health care providers are to meet the wholistic needs of clients who must make death-related decisions for themselves or those who are close to them, they must be able not only to describe the available alternatives, but also to develop skills in working with individuals and families who are facing such decisions.

HISTORICAL PERSPECTIVE

Cremation had its beginnings in the ancient Greek and Roman pagan rituals (Basevi 1920). Later, Greeks cremated their dead because of their belief that flames set the soul free (Pine 1978).

Many contemporary Eastern cultures continue to practice cremation. In some countries, cremation is a public ritual in which the body is burned on a funeral pyre that is placed on a barge in the river (Kalish 1981). The cremation of Indira Gandhi was, in fact, a national event.

In Western cultures, however, earth burial has been the more

widely accepted practice. This stems from the Judeo-Christian belief that the dead may rise again. Accordingly, the body was buried
in the earth, awaiting resurrection. Only recently has organized religion begun to accept cremation. The Roman Catholic Church main-
tained its opposition to the practice until the revision of Canon Law
by the Second Vatican Council in 1959-1963 (Ferrell 1983). Orthodox Judaism remains opposed to the practice, as do most evangelical Christian sects. The majority of Christian religions, however,
now maintain a neutral position (Minton 1981).

INCIDENCE OF CREMATION

In 1983, cremation was the method of choice for more than
249,000 representing 12.4 percent of the deaths in the United
States. This represents a significant increase, having grown from
only 2.56 percent in 1934-1938 (Staff 1984). Furthermore, the most
rapid rise in the cremation rate has occurred during the past 15
years.

In 1960, over half of the cremations in the United States took
place in the Pacific coast states (Mitford 1978). Since then, although the popularity of cremation has gradually spread to other
areas of the country, there are still almost twice as many cremations
in the Pacific states (Alaska, California, Hawaii, Oregon, and
Washington) than in any other area. In 1983, 34 percent of all cremations in the U.S. were done in those states. In contrast, the East
South Central region (Alabama, Kentucky, Mississippi, and Ten-
nessee) records less than one percent of the nation's cremations
(Staff 1984).

The significance of these figures is two-fold. First, the striking
increase in cremations in the past 25 years demonstrates that it is an
issue that the American public is confronting every day, sometimes
during the profound emotional stress that surrounds the death of a
loved one. If we, as health care providers, are to fulfill our promise
of providing holistic care, we cannot turn our backs on this issue
and thus be unable to offer the guidance and support that our clients
may need.

The second reason for addressing the data in this way is to acknowledge the geographic differences in the acceptance of crema-

tion. This may guide the emphasis placed on this aspect of the curriculum for caregivers. To be sure, educators attempt to provide health care workers who can function effectively anywhere in the nation. Nevertheless, pragmatic concern for local health needs may dictate that curricula in California, for example, place considerably more emphasis on cremation than would curricula in the East South Central region where people choose cremation for less than two percent of the deaths.

The funeral industry now encourages people to plan their funeral arrangements while they are still in good health, thereby relieving others of the need to make painful decisions at a future date. While many people have done this, planning a variety of funerals and burials, a significant number of persons have interpreted this advice slightly differently, and have prearranged their own cremation. One organization that assists with this, the National Cremation Society, signs up an average of 1,000 persons per month in Florida alone for preplanned cremation (Viqueira 1984).

REASONS FOR CHOOSING CREMATION

There are many different reasons for choosing cremation. Some of these reasons are valid and some are not. Definitive research is needed to identify the specific factors that influence the decision for cremation. Nevertheless, some factors are evident.

Minton (1981) has stated that cremation is more prevalent in urban areas where there is a concern for the need to conserve space. Indeed, for some, basic principles of land conservation become the overriding issue in the decision. The recent regulations imposed in China, requiring cremation wherever possible in order to preserve arable land, are a poignant reminder of how finite the land mass upon which we live is.

A frequently cited reason for cremation is that it is a simple, rational, and economical solution for disposal of the dead, allowing one to avoid the fuss and expense of the traditional funeral and burial. Certainly, simple cremation is substantially less expensive than an elaborate funeral. In *The American Way of Death*, however, Jessica Mitford (1978) points out that cremation can be costly when it is preceded by complete funeral services including embalming, a fancy casket, visitation, and a traditional funeral service, and is then followed by memorialization in a columbarium complete with marker and perpetual care.

Sometimes, cremation may be chosen for inappropriate reasons. The most common of these is the mistaken idea that it will spare the survivors grief, anxiety, or pain. When this is the reason for the choice, it is important to help the individual understand that loved ones will grieve regardless of the presence or absence of the dead human body, and regardless of the choice of a funeral or memorial service, earth burial or cremation. Cremation does not provide a way to avoid sorrow and grieving. When people recognize cremation as an alternative to earth burial but not as a means of avoiding grief, their decision can be rational, and options can be selected that are truly the best for themselves and their loved ones.

RELIGIOUS AND CULTURAL INFLUENCES

Although the general incidence of cremation in the United States is increasing, the stance of specific religious groups is varied. Since 1964, the Roman Catholic Church has approved of cremation, and some Roman Catholic churches now have their own columbaria to augment their cemeteries. Greek Orthodox clergy, on the other hand, are overwhelmingly opposed to cremation (Minton 1981).

Protestantism, made up of a variety of denominations, takes a variety of positions on many issues, including cremation. The great majority of Protestant churches, however, accept cremation. The resistance comes primarily from the fundamentalist and evangelical churches, but even these are not united in opposition to cremation.

Cremation is strictly forbidden in Orthodox Judaism (Goldberg 1981). Conservative Jews generally agree. The Reform Jewish faith, on the other hand, will allow cremation if it is strongly desired, although they do not encourage it (Abrams 1985).

Schneidman (1971) found that those who identified themselves as antireligious were overwhelmingly against burial. Only two percent of this group preferred earth burial in caskets, and over one-half (52 percent) wanted to be cremated.

Kalish and Reynolds (1976) found that both Mexican Americans and Blacks preferred burial to cremation at a ratio of 20:1. Conversely, over one-half of the Japanese preferred cremation.

CREMATION AND THE GRIEF PROCESS

Direct cremation is growing rapidly as the choice of many Americans today. With direct cremation, the unembalmed body is taken directly from the place of death to the crematory. It is then reduced to ashes which may be scattered at sea or in a garden or returned to the survivors for disposition as they choose. In this way, the costs of funeral director, embalming, casket, vault, and cemetery plot are avoided. Families may, of course, plan a memorial ceremony if they wish, according to their religious and philosophical preferences. In fact, the majority of cremations are followed by memorial services of some kind.

With the increase in direct cremation, there is growing concern among professionals about the effects of cremation on the grieving process. Fulton (1979) suggests that the ritual of the funeral can facilitate ventilation of profound emotions, and can assist survivors in the normal dissolution of their grief. A number of psychologists believe that viewing the dead is a significant component in the process of resolving acute grief. In addition, Fulton suggests that the experience of the funeral ceremony, whether followed by earth burial or cremation, serves to bind the survivors as they grieve, acknowledge the death, and mourn together.

It is important to recognize that the decision to cremate does not preclude the possibility of a funeral service. The two are actually separate decisions. Thus, a decision about disposition must be made by everyone, regardless of a preference for a funeral service, a memorial service, or no service. The issue is not cremation versus other means of disposition of the dead human body; rather, if cremation is chosen, the issue is what will be done with the body to meet the needs of the survivors.

With cremation, the most frequent arrangement is a memorial service, without the casket present. It is often held in a church. This brings up the highly debated issue of the importance of viewing the body. Funeral directors argue that the survivors need to see the body, to picture and remember the dead, in order to work through their grief satisfactorily. In addition, they assert that seeing the body looking attractive and at peace is therapeutic. Fulton (1979) suggests that this beautification is functional in helping the survivors accept death.

Those who disagree with this practice cite the fact that public viewing of the body and open casket ceremonies are not commonly practiced in Jewish funerals, yet it has not been determined that Jews have more difficulty resolving their grief than Christians who may have both public viewing during "visitation" and open casket funerals. Corr (1979) questions whether it is desirable to view the person as though sleeping, but restored to life, for this does not convey the reality of death, and Lamm (1969) suggests that the acceptance of the death is more difficult if the survivors see the dead as if still alive.

It is important to many survivors to have a place to go to remember the dead. To fill this need, it is not unusual for a cemetery to provide a columbarium, where urns containing cremated remains ("cremains," as they are now called in the trade) can be placed in niches, memorial plaques can be affixed, and the family can visit the site just as they can an earth grave. In fact, some churches are beginning to provide columbaria, in addition to cemeteries, for their members.

Another alternative is to bury the cremains in the family plot, beside or on top of the caskets of other family members. Scattering the cremains further decreases cost by eliminating the need for an urn, a niche in a columbarium, and a memorial plaque. However, this can also eliminate the memorialization that is important to many. Furthermore, there is then no place that survivors can visit, and this activity is emotionally important to some persons.

ROLE OF THE HEALTH CARE PROFESSIONAL

McCorkle (1982) suggests that nurses encourage families to make some decisions before the death occurs, in order to ease the pain and pressure of such decisions when it may be more difficult. The health care provider, through sensitive intervention, can ensure that clients make informed choices and that they receive the support they need as they make those choices.

Preplanning one's own funeral or other after-death arrangements affords a dying person some control over those final plans and can be helpful for the terminally ill person who feels a lack of control over his or her destiny. In this situation, the care giver can help the individual to consider the needs of the survivors.

Health care providers must maintain a sensitivity to the client's and family's religious and cultural traditions, and tailor the interventions accordingly. For example, knowledge of Orthodox Jewish teachings would dissuade the care giver from initiating a discussion with someone of that faith of the pros and cons of cremation or of viewing of the body.

A problem can occur when one person in a family wants cremation but another does not. This disagreement may occur between husband and wife or between parent and child. The health care worker may be able to assist the persons involved to discuss their feelings openly and to come to a decision that is mutually acceptable.

CREMATION-RELATED ISSUES

If the health care provider is to act as a client advocate, he or she must be knowledgeable about cremation. Certainly, good health care does not include teaching every client "everything you always wanted to know about cremation, but were afraid to ask." However, the care giver must be prepared to offer information when needed, to correct misinformation, and to base interventions on sound knowledge. The client will thereby be supported in making his or her own best decision.

A basic knowledge of such things as legal issues and common practices will allow the health care professional to intervene when needed to correct misconceptions and assist with planning. For example, a new Federal Trade Commission ruling requires that prices for funeral services must be itemized, that permission of next-of-kin must be obtained before embalming, and that prices must be quoted over the phone if requested.

Embalming is an issue that is often misunderstood. Although it provides temporary preservation of the body and is therefore helpful for public viewing, it is not required by law. Thus, the health care provider can act as a client advocate for persons desiring direct cremation. These persons can be helped to understand that embalming may be an unnecessary service, and expense, which they can refuse.

A related issue is that of the container for the body. When a person requests cremation, the law does not require purchase of a casket. In fact, some of the heavier metal caskets pose specific problems in cremation (Mitford 1978). Information about alternatives and common practice can be helpful to the client who is wrestling with this decision.

Information about the containers selected most frequently for cremation appears in a 1982 survey of crematories in the United States (Staff 1982). Figures represent all cremations, whether or not accompanied by a traditional funeral service or a memorial service. The survey shows that in 58.5 percent of all cremations, a cardboard box was the container used. If the health care provider is aware that the cardboard box is the container of choice in the majority of cremations, he or she may be able to use this information in reassuring and supporting the individual who is torn between the conflicting emotions of concern for simplicity and economy, and a desire to provide the "best" for his or her loved one.

In some states, the body must be held for 48 hours after death before being cremated. This waiting period prevents immediate cremation, in case an autopsy or other examination should be needed. Other states, however, have shorter waiting periods, or even no wait at all except for the death certificate and coroner's permit. Thus, it behooves the care giver to know the local requirements in order to provide knowledgeable guidance and support to families.

CREMATION IN THE THANATOLOGY CURRICULUM

Including Cremation in the Curriculum

Knott (1979) proposes three major goals for death education: information sharing, personal values clarification, and the development of coping skills.

The first of Knott's goals is information sharing. The cremation information that is important was suggested earlier and includes the following: economic issues, needs of survivors, separation of the funeral/memorial service decision from the decision about disposition of the body, effects on the grieving process, religious and cultural issues, people's attitudes and values, alternatives for memorialization, alternatives for containers, Federal Trade Commission rulings, and legal issues of embalming, use of caskets, and waiting periods. This knowledge prepares the health care professional to provide whatever information the client may need, and to correct misinformation before the client acts on it. In this way, the health care provider can help the client to make the best decision.

The second goal is personal values clarification. Cremation is a topic fraught with emotion, related partly to misunderstandings and partly to individual attitudes and experiences. If health care workers are to provide support to persons making decisions about cremation, those care givers must first clarify and come to terms with their own personal values related to this practice.

The third of Knott's suggested goals relates to coping behaviors and includes problem-solving skills. In order to assist clients who are deciding about disposition of the body after death, health care providers must first have an understanding of coping behaviors and develop their own problem-solving skills. This is particularly important for our students, since American youth today typically have had no experience with death and mourning and therefore have not had the opportunity for this kind of growth.

Placement of Cremation in the Curriculum

The curricula of some schools of nursing, medicine, and related health professions include a variety of specific courses in thanatology. The content related to cremation could appropriately be addressed in several of the courses. For example, communication skills for initiating and following through with a discussion of plans for disposition of the body could be addressed in a course on communication skills for care givers in death and dying. Similarly, factual knowledge about cremation could be addressed in a course dealing with funeral customs and practices, and a discussion of the potential effects of various choices on the grieving process could be addressed in a course on grief and mourning.

Not many curricula, however, provide a comprehensive roster of thanatology courses from which the student can select courses with a variety of foci. More often, one single course addresses death and dying. In this case, the issues addressed in this paper should be included in that one course. This content related to cremation would logically be included as part of the section that addresses funerals, with cremation presented as an alternative to the more traditional methods of disposition of the body.

Some curricula do not include any courses devoted exclusively to thanatology. The curricula of schools of nursing, medicine, and related health professions today are overcrowded with the exploding technology, ethical issues, and economics of today's rapidly changing health care system. This does not necessitate the abandonment of thanatology concepts, however. Many courses in health care deal with death and dying when they discuss issues in medical health care, surgical health care, care of the acute and chronically ill, gerontology, oncology, etc. Content related to cremation can be effectively integrated into these courses as they address providing support to clients and their families who are confronted with death.

Although actual discussions of health care providers' roles related to cremation are rarely found in health care curricula, the literature has begun to recognize the need for courses to address the alternatives available to clients. Swain and Cowles (1982) describe an interdisciplinary death education course that they have developed at the University of Wisconsin-Milwaukee School of Nursing. In this course, they provide material on postdeath activities, including alternatives to the traditional funeral and disposal of the body. In fact, one of the objectives of this course is that the student "describes typical steps to be taken for making funeral arrangements and burial in our society and the alternatives available."

Ulin (1977) suggested that the thanatology curriculum must include such issues as the nature of funeral options and the value of choosing early. In his prototype for a course in death and dying, one objective involves identifying alternatives available to the public related to funeral procedures and practices, including the disposition of the body. He further asserted that the costs associated with death are an important part of death education.

McCorkle (1982) makes a similar suggestion when discussing a course in death and dying designed for graduate nursing students. McCorkle asserts that nurses should develop skills that include the ability to assist with the plans and needs of the family after death, including funeral arrangements.

Communication Skills Needed

The development of effective communication skills is important in the thanatology curriculum. In assessing the helpfulness of various communication techniques, Myrick and Wittmer (1980) developed a probability continuum of facilitative responses. They identified low facilitative responses as advice/evaluation, interpretation/analysis, and reassurance/support. These verbal behaviors are often accompanied by the best of intentions but fall short of being helpful to the grieving individual. On the other hand, responses involving open questioning, clarification/summary, and those responses that focus on feelings were perceived as highly facilitative. An understanding of this continuum and its implications can be helpful to the student who is attempting to develop communication skills for addressing such a sensitive issue as cremation.

CONCLUSION

In "Death Education for All," Knott (1979) asserted, ". . . no other single target area for thanatology has the potential to alter societal views of mortality as profoundly and immediately as does effective death education for medical care givers." And just what is effective death education? Jeanne Quint Benoliel (1982) states, "Death education for nurses and physicians requires more than an opportunity to become sensitive to personal reactions — though this aspect is important. It requires opportunity to grapple with the complexities of choice and decision affecting the lives of others in profound ways."

Persons in the health care professions deal daily with clients faced with the question of determining the means of disposition of the body after death. If professional care givers are to assist clients in reaching the best decisions and then to support them in those decisions, the care givers must first have an understanding of the factors that may influence that decision. Only then can they assist and support the client who struggles with decisions that are irrevocable and may have long-term effects on his or her own emotional and psychological well-being and that of his or her loved ones.

Statistics demonstrate the increasing acceptance of cremation in this country. Nevertheless, there exists a lack of awareness of its various implications, both among the public and among health care providers. A study done by Garman and Kidd (1983) found people largely unprepared for their own funerals, despite the current trend toward more candid talk about death and dying and despite the attempts of the funeral industry to educate the general public and to promote planning. Thus it is all too likely that people may come to the threshold of a death experience, their own or that of a loved one, without adequate knowledge upon which to base a rational decision. In such a time of emotional stress, the individual will be in even greater need of professional guidance and support in order to make decisions with which he or she can be comfortable. Surely it is the responsibility of those who design thanatology curricula to address this need in concrete ways.

REFERENCES

Abrams, J. M. February 26, 1985. Personal Communication.

Basevi, H. (1920). *The Burial of the Dead*. London: Routledge and Sons.

Benoliel, J. C. (1982). "Introduction to the special Issue." *Death Education*, 5: ix-x.

Corr, C. A. (1979). "Living with the changing face of death." In H. Wass (Ed.). *Dying: Facing the Facts*, 44-72. Washington: Hemisphere.

Ferrell, D. G. (1983). "Implications of cremation for grief adjustment." *National Reporter*, 6(7): 2-6.

Fulton, R. H. (1979). "Death and the funeral in contemporary society." In H. Wass, (Ed.). *Dying: Facing the Facts*, 236-255. Washington: Hemisphere.

Garman, E. T. and Kidd, C. A. (1983). "Consumer preparedness, knowledge, and opinions about practices and regulations of the funeral industry." *Death Education*. 6: 341-352.

Goldberg, H. S. (1981). "Funerals and bereavement rituals of Kota indians and Orthodox Jews." *Omega*. 12: 117-128.

Kalish, R. A. (1981). *Death, Grief, and Caring Relationships*. Monterrey, CA: Brooks/Cole.

Kalish, R. A. and Reynolds, D. K. (1976). *Death and Ethnicity: A Psychocultural Study*. Los Angeles: University of Southern California Press.

Knott, J. E. (1979). "Death education for all." In H. Wass (Ed.). *Dying: Facing the Facts*, 385-403. Washington: Hemisphere.

Lamm, M. (1969). *The Jewish Way in Death and Mourning*. New York: Jonathon David.

McCorkle, R. (1982). "Death education for advanced nursing practice." *Death Education*, *5*, 347-361.

Minton, F. (1981). "Clergy views of funeral practices (Part One)." *National Reporter*, *4*(4), 2-5.

Mitford, J. (1978). *The American Way of Death*. New York: Simon and Schuster.

Myrick, R. and Wittmer, J. (1980). *Facilitative Teaching: Theory and Practice* (2nd ed.). Minneapolis: Educational Media Corporation.

Pine, V. R. (1978). "The care of the dead: A historical portrait." In R. Fulton, E. Markusen, G. Owen, and J. L. Scheiber (Eds.). *Death and Dying: Challenge and Change*, 272-278. Reading, Mass.: Addison-Wesley.

Schneidman, E. S. (1971). "You and death." *Psychology Today*, *5*(1), 43-45, 74-80.

Staff. (1984). "Cremation historical figures: 1876 on." *The Cremationist*.

Staff. (1982). Joint CANA/CMA Container and Disposition Survey. *CANA News Report*.

Swain, H. L. and Cowles, K. V. (1982). "Interdisciplinary death education in a nursing school." *Death Education*, *5*, 297-315.

Ulin, R. O. (1977). *Death and Dying Education*. Washington, D.C.: National Education Association.

Viqueira, J. December 28, 1984. Personal communication.

Death Education Changes
Coping to Confidence

Pat Babcock

Death has been identified as one of the last taboo subjects of the current generation (Vickery 1974). The curricula of schools of nursing have not treated the subject of death and dying as taboo, but have introduced the topic as a one hour lecture in post-mortem care. The physiologic manifestations of death are routinely taught in nursing courses, but the emotional needs of the dying person receive minimal attention.

Nursing school curricula have emphasized the life-saving skills of nursing practice. Priority has been given to the recovery and discharge of the patient or to assistance in the adjustment to changes in daily living. Little emphasis has been placed on the ethical and legal considerations of nursing practice related to death and dying. The emotional needs of the dying patient were frequently avoided due to a feeling of inadequacy on the part of the nurse when death was imminent.

The lack of course offerings relative to death and dying is distressing when death provokes fear and a state of helplessness for individuals responsible for the care of the dying patient (Wagner 1964). Classroom desensitization was planned prior to the clinical experience at one university to assist the student more effectively in dealing with the needs of the patient and family. Classroom discussions and assigned readings broadened the knowledge base of the students. The ventilation of death fears and concerns which had been internalized over the years were facilitated by the classroom exercises (Wagner 1964).

A study of nursing students and graduate nurses (Golub and Reznikoff 1971) was conducted to test the difference in attitudes toward the influence of psychological factors upon death, autopsy, and treatment of the seriously ill. Conclusions reached were that nursing education related to death and dying created an awareness of the importance of psychological factors influencing attitudes toward death, and that those attitudes then remain stable throughout the career of the nurse.

Lester, Getty, and Kneisl (1974) investigated undergraduate nursing students, graduate nursing students, and nursing faculty to determine if fears of death and dying would decrease with additional education in the area of thanatology. The results of the study indicated that fears related to death and dying decreased with more education except for junior undergraduate students and first year graduate students (Lester, Getty, and Kneisl 1974).

Other research which emphasized the importance of thanatology courses in the nursing curriculum was that of Yeaworth, Kapp, and Winget (1974). A questionnaire designed to measure attitudes toward death and dying was administered to freshmen and senior students. The senior students demonstrated greater acceptance of feelings, more open communication, and broader flexibility in relating to dying patients and their relatives. The overall findings of the research suggested that important changes in attitudes relative to death and dying can result from nursing education if thanatology courses are required.

Death education provides the student the opportunity to investigate and begin to comprehend personal concerns of death and dying. A course in death education would include a background of cultural and social values that have historically influenced the acceptance of death as a normal state. An educational experience would be provided in the conceptualization of decision making and practice (Benoliel 1982).

In spite of the publication of many studies demonstrating the importance of a required course in thanatology in the nursing curriculum, there are few programs meeting the need. The Thrush and Paulus Survey (1978) reported that only 5 percent of the 205 schools of nursing surveyed in the United States required a course in death and dying and 39.5 percent indicated that an elective course was available.

The paucity of thanatology courses has resulted in inconsistent interactions between the nurse and the dying patient. The extended life span of the individual and the marked reduction in childhood deaths due to infectious diseases have created a death-free environment for many student nurses. Due to the migration trends of our society, many families are located a great distance from parents and grandparents. The physical distance can also create an emotional distancing which results in less grief experience when death occurs.

In addition to an absence of the death of significant others in their lives, student nurses may only rarely be assigned to dying patients during clinical rotation. With the minimum integration of the subject of death and dying throughout the curriculum, the student has a limited knowledge of the physical and emotional needs of the dying patient. If the student nurse does not have the responsibility for the care of dying patients, he or she will not be able to take advantage of the emotional support from the faculty member sponsoring the clinical laboratory.

Therapeutic interventions for a dying patient must be learned just as any other technical skill. The mastery of specified technical skills must be achieved prior to the completion of a semester in order to meet the critical criteria of the course. Clinical interventions related to meeting the emotional needs of the dying person are not included in the required critical criteria of a course.

The void created by the minimal lecture content (one hour in fundamentals and approximately two hours in psychiatric mental health nursing) of the nursing curriculum at Purdue University North Central indicated a need for a course in thanatology. Some postconference time was utilized to discuss the process of death and the needs of a dying patient and family, but this time was episodic rather than an integrated part of study.

A course was developed to meet the needs of the nursing students and the graduates of the program. The class closes early in the registration period due to the popularity of the topic. The elective offering is a three-credit-hour course and is open to all university students each spring semester. A requirement of nursing fundamentals was required for the first four years the course was offered, but this prerequisite was eliminated due to frequent requests for enrollment from students enrolled in other programs at the university.

The primary purpose of the course is to increase the awareness of a professional regarding personal concerns toward death in order to provide more effective care of the dying patient. A conceptual understanding of thanatology is gained by the study of medical, social, religious, psychological, and legal aspects of death as it pertains to the care giver, client, and society. The course is divided into lectures for a theoretical background and small group seminars. The small group seminars allow the student the opportunity to explore and verbalize personal concerns and/or values regarding death. The student who successfully completes this course will:

1. Have increased personal awareness of individuals' concerns about death.
2. Have assessed his or her personal philosophy and attitudes toward death and dying.
3. Have recognized the role which values play in determining life and death styles of individuals.
4. Have examined the complexities involved in modern definitions of death.
5. Have critically evaluated ethical issues related to the dying persons.
6. Have recognized developmental levels which require consideration in planning intervention.
7. Have formulated constructive plans for his or her own or a relative's death in terms of personal, social, and legal aspects.
8. Be able to identify the functions of rituals associated with death, funerals, and mourning.
9. Be able to describe normal and abnormal reactions to bereavement seen in the grief process.
10. Have examined death-related issues including euthanasia, sudden infant death syndrome, suicide, and treatment of terminally ill clients.
11. Have developed basic competencies in supporting a terminally ill client and/or a bereaved family member or significant other.

12. Be able to identify common clues indicative of potential suicidal behavior.
13. Be knowledgeable about cultural and religious views concerning death.
14. Be able to evaluate alternatives to hospitalization during the final stage of life.
15. Have increased ability to recognize "burnout" in themselves or colleagues.
16. Be able to identify the need for "support systems" for professionals who work with terminally ill clients.

The content of the course was planned to provide a broad-based knowledge of thanatology. It includes:

Unit I Death and Contemporary Society

    a. Attitudes Toward Death
    b. Personal Death Concerns
    c. Historical Overview
    d. Encounters with Death

Unit II Death and Ritual

    a. Significance of the Funeral
    b. Religious Aspects of Death

Unit III Death and Health Care

    a. Definitions of Death
    b. Physical Aspects of Dying
    c. Medical, Legal, and Philosophical Considerations

Unit IV Death Resulting from Suicide or Murder

Unit V Stages of Dying and Grief

    a. Psychological Coping Patterns
    b. Dealing with Death: The Child, the Adolescent, and the Adult

Unit VI Right To Die: Professional Concerns and Issues

a. Euthanasia
b. Current Legislation
c. Support Groups

Unit VII Principles of Intervention

a. Professional Roles
b. Coping Strategies/Ego Mechanisms
c. Communication Skills

Unit VIII Personal and Societal Choices

a. Recognition of Personal Death Concerns
b. Hospice
c. Wills, Organ Transplants

Outside speakers are invited to share their expertise with the students. A rabbi, a priest, a minister, and a bishop in the Church of Jesus Christ of Latter Day Saints explain the religious beliefs of their faiths. A hospice representative presents an overview of the program and shows the film, "Day by Day." Representatives from the local organization of Compassionate Friends provide a panel discussion followed by a question and answer period.

Various filmstrips, movies, tapes, and music are also used to enhance the lecture portion of the course. Small group exercises have been developed for role playing. Various clinical interventions and communication skills are practiced during the seminar time. Course evaluations at the end of the term have expressed positive feedback for skills learned and utilized during this portion of the class.

The course is designed so the student will begin to recognize the influence of society, ethnic and cultural heritage, and past experiences on their personal death concerns. A modified contract system is used for the course. The student decides what activities will be undertaken to earn the desired grade. Personal growth in the area of thanatology and increased confidence in the care of the dying patient and his or her family are the goals of the course. The goals are achieved more readily if an experiential approach is utilized instead of a didactic one. Regular class attendance and participation are necessary if this end is to be met.

The funeral home visits have been very popular. Some students have never been inside a funeral home and have had many misconceptions regarding the atmosphere and functions. Several of the students have contracted for their funeral arrangements following the visit. Many more have planned their own funeral services as a creative project.

The purpose of creative projects is to encourage the student to investigate an area of thanatology which would most effectively meet a need of the student. Creative projects have ranged from tombstone etching, a study of Indian funeral customs (following a local archeology excavation which uncovered Indian artifacts), to a series of interviews with family members who survived the massacre of a family unit.

Keeping a diary has been beneficial for many of the students. Thoughts of death have been much more frequent and random at the beginning of class, but committing thoughts and feelings to paper have helped to clarify them.

The contract for the course follows:

CONTRACT

Thanatology 355

CONTRACT GRADE SYSTEM: Thanatology will operate on a modified Contract Grading System. This type of system puts the burden of grades on the student. All students are required to complete the *core* activities (possible points = 60). Each student (to meet his or her particular needs) can choose alternate learning tasks to complete the requirements of the grade desired. NOTE: Please cushion yourself with *more* points than necessary for the grade you want, as the points given are the maximum, not necessarily what you will achieve.

A. Core Requirements: *REQUIRED OF ALL STUDENTS.*

   1. Short paper, 5-10 double-spaced pages. This paper should analyze an issue in thanatology. In the analysis, note various possible arguments which could be advanced; then argue for a position of your own. *20 points* possible. (Due April 17.)
   2. Field trip to funeral home and personal funeral cost sheet. *10 points.*
   3. Attendance and participation. *25 points.*

B. Optional Activities. *YOUR CHOICE FOR CONTRACT.*

   1. Completion of a creative project dealing with some aspect of death or dying that will significantly add to our understanding of these phenomena. *20 points possible.* (Will be evaluated on the basis of appropriateness, significance, innovative ideas and insights.)
   2. Choose an area in thanatology that is unresolved and cite various possible consequences of at least three possible solutions to the issue. Include the areas of *Law, Sociology, Psychology, Medicine, Theology, Science* (if applicable). *10 points possible.*
   3. Abstracts from periodicals—nursing, medical, psychology, sociology—which deal with thanatology. (Will be evaluated on clarity, insight and appropriateness.) *5 points possible per abstract.* Maximum of four abstracts.
   4. Prepare an oral presentation on a particular issue in thanatology to be given in class. (Could be done as a group using role playing, etc.). *10 points possible.*
   5. Keep a diary of your feelings regarding the subject of death. This will include personal and academic experiences and feelings. It will be discussed with instructor three or four times per semester. *20 points possible.*

GRADING SCALE:

$$93 - 100 = A$$
$$85 - 92 = B$$
$$75 - 84 = C$$

70 − 74 = D

Below 70 = F

The class offers an opportunity for students to confront fears of death and dying. These include both fears of personal death and fears of not being able to meet the emotional needs of a dying patient. Several students have verbalized a feeling of vacillation between merely coping with the needs of a dying patient and avoiding both the patient and family. This inconsistency was one of the motivating factors for enrolling in the course. Other students have stated that they have unresolved grief which is blocking their personal and professional growth.

Approximately half of the students are at the undergraduate level and half are graduates of an associate degree program. Blending of the experiences of the undergraduate and graduate students have enhanced the quality of the course content.

The first lecture of the course establishes the ground rules for the semester. A nonjudgmental and relaxed atmosphere encourages open interaction between students and faculty. The degree of confidence gained from the course will vary with each individual as will the time required to reach each plateau of comprehension and assimilation of facts. The freedom to express any concerns or beliefs facilitates the examination of death concerns. Differences of opinion encourage further investigation of personal beliefs.

Another positive aspect of the course is the ripple effect which extends to family, significant others, or friends. One of my students had been unable to establish any communication with her husband following the death of a twin son. Nine years had passed since the death, but he was still unable to confront the issue. By the end of the semester lines of communication were opened so the death could be discussed. In addition, her husband helped to plan both their funeral services and designed a marker for their graves. Positive examples of application of knowledge and insight occur each semester.

The knowledge gained from a class in death education is being incorporated into life situations. One of the registered nurse students who took the class saw a need for a grief team in the hospital where she worked. A literature search was done to determine if any information was available on the subject, but none was found. The instructor of the course met with the nurses who had taken the course and with the director of staff education to establish guidelines and goals for the concept of a grief team. The concept was implemented and was very successful in meeting the needs of the institution, causing the nurse to write an article on the topic which was later accepted for publication in a nursing journal.

The role of the nurse is rapidly changing. We are no longer the handmaidens of the physician, but are intelligent professionals who are attempting to implement wholistic nursing care for the patient. One method of meeting this goal is to meet the emotional needs of all patients, but in particular those of the dying patient. Death education is an effective method of changing mere coping to confidence on the part of the nurse.

REFERENCES

Benoliel, J. Q. (Ed.) (1982). *Death Education for the Health Profession*. Washington: Hemisphere Publishing Corporation.

Golub, S. and Reznikoff, N. (1971). "Attitudes toward death." *Nursing Research, 20*, 503-508.

Lester, D., Getty, C., & Kneisl, C. R. (1974). "Attitudes of nursing students and nursing faculty toward death." *Nursing Research, 23*, 50-53.

Thrush, J.C., & Paulus, G. S. (1979). "The availability of education on death and dying: A survey of U.S. nursing schools." *Death Education, 3*(2), 131-42.

Vickery, K. (1974). "Medical survival—The press, the public, the profession, and the patient." *Royal Society of Health, 94*, 118-23.

Wagner, B. (1964). "Teaching students to work with the dying." *American Journal of Nursing, 64*, 128.

Yeaworth, R. C., Kapp, F. T., & Winget, C. (1974). "Attitudes of nursing students toward the dying patient." *Nursing Research, 23*, 20-24.

The L.P.N.:
Ability to Deliver Care
to the Terminally Ill

Catherine O. D'Amico

Practical nursing's roots are in caring for the chronically ill in the home. The first practical nursing program was established in 1893 by the YMCA in Brooklyn for just that purpose. The success of this course inspired the development of others. The curriculum included cooking, care of the home, dietetics, simple science, and nursing procedures. However, the public at this time had no knowledge of the level of education of the person hired to care for an ill family member in the home.

Fifty years later, in the 1940s, the title Licensed Practical/Vocational Nurse was established. Throughout the 1940s practices to evaluate learning and curriculum through accrediting agencies and state-administered licensing exams were set in place. The L.P.N. was now prepared to function side-by-side with the professional (registered) nurse and independently with little supervision from physicians or other nurses. The characteristics of practical nursing education are now defined by the National League for Nursing as:

> programs . . . designed to meet the need in nursing services for a nurse who will share in the giving of direct care to patients. They are intended for individuals who will find satisfaction in (1) performing nursing functions consistent with short-term preparation and (2) practicing nursing within a limited range of patient care situations. (Beaver, Lynch and Micali 1980, p. 7)

Educational experiences are designed to achieve these goals. The situations provided allow each student to learn the nursing of patients in selected situations and to learn direct patient care. Basic

45

information in the biological and behavioral sciences is still the root of the curriculum. Care of patients of all age levels and socioeconomic groups, and with common deviations in their health, are basic within all practical nursing programs. Practical nursing education, as it exists today, teaches the graduate to relate concepts to care, not just to memorize facts (D'Amico 1965). Although the practical nurse may learn to care for the client with cancer who is 40 years old, she can relate the concepts associated with this diagnosis and the concepts associated with growth and development to care for clients of school age and old age with a similar diagnosis.

The following concepts and expected outcomes of behavior are consistent throughout most practical nursing programs. It is these concepts and outcomes that make the practical nurse an ideal care giver to the terminally ill client. Beaver et al. (1980) give the following outline:

CONCEPTS

The Practical Nurse

1. Assesses current and potential health status. Using the nursing process, the graduate focuses on alleviating, minimizing, or preventing problems. She maintains and promotes her patients' health.
2. Maintains a nurse/patient relationship and professional relationships by utilizing an effective communication system.
3. Manages her own actions and plans and organizes patient activities in a structured setting.
4. Utilizes knowledge from the physical and behavioral sciences as sources for making practical nursing decisions.
5. Accepts individual responsibility for practical nursing actions.

EXPECTED BEHAVIOR OUTCOMES AND COMPETENCIES

The Practical Nurse

1. Contributes to the identification of basic physical, emotional, and cultural needs of the patient.
2. Identifies and uses basic communication techniques.
3. Interviews patients to obtain specific information.

4. Identifies overt needs of the patient and family (significant others).
5. Makes observations and reports them to the appropriate team member (R.N., physician).
6. Identifies appropriate resources in other agencies (requests assistance of physical therapist, dietician, or social worker through the R.N. or physician).
7. Safely provides basic therapeutic and preventive nursing procedures (incorporating principles of physical and behavioral sciences).
8. Applies basic communication techniques.
9. Demonstrates health teaching during routine care.
10. Shows respect for the dignity of individuals.
11. Evaluates, with guidance, the care given assigned patients and makes appropriate changes.

Throughout the concepts and outcomes, the author makes references to the practical nurse's ability to give physical care, provide emotional support, and recognize and communicate change to others, i.e., the professional nurse and the physician. Throughout the educational experience, the practical nurse defers to these professionals for support and guidance in changing the care required. She is consistently given opportunities to give physical care and emotional support in situations where she must recognize and report change in the patient's health status. While she is not prohibited from changing daily routine, decisions about intensifying care beyond providing safety and comfort are made by the professionals.

The emphasis on communication and recognition of change are critical in the care of the terminally ill. Recognition and communication of change provide the impetus for increasing comfort through other physical care and through chemical methods. The practical nurse has been taught to deliver this care but she leaves the decision of when to do so to others.

Within a structured framework, the practical nurse can observe the patient and gather information to provide necessary care for comfort in the end stages of life or when prolonging life, if that is the choice of the patient. Under the guidance of a professional nurse or physician, the practical nurse can collect data, so that the health professionals can collaborate on changes and/or maintenance of care.

This structured framework need not be a hospital or nursing home setting. The practical nurse can provide care in the home as well, whenever lines of communication to professional sources are available.

The L.P.N.'s level of education is ideally suited to the care of the terminally ill, whose status may change slowly. Care may remain very similar over long periods of time, but she has, at the same time, the skills necessary to communicate subtle, as well as acute, changes and to seek guidance in handling these situations. Her license provides her with the means to provide comfort by chemical as well as physical means. Unlike the nurse's aide, the practical nurse's training in the physical and behavioral sciences enables her to observe subtle change and initiate care and communications to deal with that change. She can provide information to significant others and to the client which is realistic rather than optimistic when there is little hope or pessimistic without reason.

The practical nurse assures the patient and those close to him or her that a particular level of skill and education has been achieved. Dying is frequently a slow and costly process. Competent care provided at a reasonable cost is yet another reason for utilizing the practical nurse in a home care setting.

The population presently seeking practical nursing education is frequently from minority groups. These people are mature and usually older than the traditional 4-year college graduate. They frequently come to this education with considerable experience with dying and the rituals which surround it in their own culture and in others. They have more life experiences, which enables them to cope with the frustration, anxiety, doubts, and fears of the dying client and his or her significant others. Maturity and experience assist them in their communication with the patient and the professionals who designate the care.

Within her education, the practical nurse deals with her feelings about death and dying. Through core curricula which contain sociological and psychological theory — appropriate to a 1-year curriculum — death and the grieving process are explored (Kübler-Ross 1975). Ethical issues of dignity, death with dignity, and bereavement are discussed. This permits the students to exchange the feelings and cultural mores which surround death, dying, and bereavement. The exploration of various practices assists students in accepting and respecting the practices of others as they examine their own feelings about how they would wish themselves or their families to be treated when death is a predictable outcome (Stanley 1980).

The practical nurse, because of the emphasis on clinical practice in her educational background, utilizing the underlying principles of the physical, behavioral, and social sciences, provides care which anticipates and meets the needs of the dying patient and his or her significant others in the hospital, in the skilled nursing and health-related facility, or in the home care setting.

REFERENCES

Beaver, K., Lynch, S. and Micali, J. (1980). *Practical Nursing: Curricula and Competencies*. New York: National League for Nursing.

D'Amico, C. 0. (1965). *Practical Nursing Education – A Guide to Curriculum Development*. New York: National Association for Practical Nurse Education and Service.

Kübler-Ross, E. (1975). "Preface: A journey into the realm of death and growth." In *Death – The Final Stage of Growth*. Englewood Cliffs, N.J.: Prentice-Hall, Inc.

Stanley, Sr. Theresa (1980). "Ethics as a component of the curriculum." *Ethical Issues in Nursing and Nursing Education*. New York: National League for Nursing.

The Near-Death Experience:
Implications for Nursing Education

Mary Dee McEvoy

Topics related to death and dying are included in the curriculum of programs in nursing in several ways: through the systematic integration of specifically designed courses; by happenstance, when the topic becomes of concern to students; as a specific course, either required or as an elective; or as a postconference topic of discussion after the clinical experience. Regardless of the method, areas of discussion generally include paradigms of dying, communication, funeral practices, cultural implications, personal beliefs and attitudes, and legal and ethical issues. Another topic, the Near-Death Experience, is imperative to those courses examining the nature of the dying experience, that is, "What is it like to be dying?"

Recently, a variety of experiences occurring during sudden death, termed the Near-Death Experience (NDE), have been described. The topic is familiar due to the popular 1975 best seller by Raymond Moody, *Life After Life*. The NDE includes subjective reports of people who have come close to death and were subsequently resuscitated. During resuscitation, a pattern of experiences has been reported, including a feeling of peace and quiet, an out-of-the-body experience, entering a dark tunnel, seeing a being of light, and experiencing a panoramic review of life. Many people dismissed Moody's book, calling it too subjective with no consideration for systematic inquiry. However, subsequent examination of the topic, using structured interview methods and statistical analysis (Ring 1980; Sabom 1982), did not refute Moody's work. Indeed, case studies continue to be collected at a steady pace (Bush 1983; Green 1983; Ring 1981; Greyson and Stevenson 1980). While these

51

reports follow a consistent pattern, accounts do vary in terms of the depth of the experience.

One helpful way of examining the NDE is provided in the work of Greyson (1983). His research uncovered four predominant components; cognitive, affective, paranormal, and transcendental. The cognitive aspect includes the accentuation of both time and thoughts, a panoramic review of life, and increased understanding. The affective component includes feelings of peace and joy, a sense of harmony with the universe, and a feeling of being surrounded by a brilliant light. The paranormal component includes the out-of-the-body experience, vivid sensations, and a perception of scenes from the future. Finally, the transcendental component includes entering an unearthly world, encountering a mystical being, seeing spirits, and encountering a border.

Some aspects of the NDE have also been reported by persons dying over a long period, rather than from an acute illness. Relating to the affective and cognitive components, the literature on the dying experience generally contradicts the reports of peace and calm, reporting instead feelings of anxiety and depression (Hinton 1963). Osis (1961) and Osis and Heraldsson (1977) conducted interviews of physicians and nurses regarding the dying experience. Their retrospective study gives evidence of the paranormal and transcendental components, reporting that terminally ill people have experienced visions of religious figures, visions of an other-worldly place, an out-of-the-body experience, and an elevation of mood. Also, almost any health care provider can give anecdotal reports relating to these experiences. This author recalls one woman seeing bright lights and religious figures prior to death. Frequently, we see patients reaching their hands toward something or someone just before death and also patients calling out the names of deceased friends and relatives. These reports, although anecdotal, can be examined in relation to the paranormal component.

The questions now, of course, are "What of it?" "Why should we be interested in this?" Or, more specifically, "Why should we teach this?" The answers rest in two areas: individual responses to the NDE by those who experience it, and the interest of the popular press in anything related to the paranormal component. People who have experienced NDEs generally report a favorable response to them. They become more religious, in the general sense of the term, and they report a decrease in the fear of death and an increase in the belief in life after death (Sabom 1982). They also report a transformation in their value systems and an increase in concern for others (Flynn 1982). Interestingly, although this response is positive, patients were reluctant to talk about their experience with health care personnel for fear of being considered crazy. Indeed, this is the crux of the matter for educators, for, when they were given the opportunity to discuss their experience, patients universally said they felt better. They indicated relief in knowing that others have had similar experiences, and discussion helped them clarify their own feelings about the experience. It would seem, then, if we as nurses are to assist people in their responses to health and illness, we need to be knowledgeable about the NDE and its impact on people's lives.

Another matter for consideration is the abundance of articles in the popular press regarding life after death. Experiences such as the NDE are frequently cited as evidence for life after death, although in reality, they do not provide such evidence. Many of us have stood in lines at the supermarket and noted a variety of headlines in papers such as *The National Enquirer*. These sensational articles can frighten people, cause disbelief in any unusual phenomenon or even, at the other extreme, lead them to expect the experience themselves. If a dying person does see religious figures, the family may think the person crazy. Or, alternatively, the dying person and the family may actually think they *should* be seeing religious figures and wonder why they aren't. In either case, the nurse must know about the reality of the NDE and its effects. Hence, the topic is not only appropriate but indeed imperative in any thanatology curriculum.

Given that the NDE is appropriate to a thanatology curriculum, let us consider some objectives and teaching methods. Learning objectives should address knowledge and understanding of the NDE, and also, because nursing is a practical profession, the more pragmatic way of talking with patients about it. Here are some possibilities:

1. The student should have an understanding of the nature of the near-death experience and its subsequent impact on patients.
2. The student should have an understanding of his or her personal beliefs and attitudes relating to the paranormal and transcendental aspects of the NDE.
3. The student should develop strategies to assist the patient in discussion of the NDE.

Teaching methods could include didactic presentations and video presentations. The International Association for Near-Death Studies in Storrs, Connecticut produces some video tapes of patient reports of NDEs. In terms of texts specific to the NDE, *Life at Death* by Kenneth Ring (1980) and *Recollections of Death* by Michael Sabom (1982) are the most scientific presentations of the subject. Sabom's chapter on the causes of the experience is excellent. Schneidman (1976) in his popular text, *Death: Current Perspectives* and Kastenbaum (1979) in *Between Life and Death* have chapters that contain some aspects of the NDE.

As Greyson and Stevenson (1980) state, "The investigation of near-death experiences may contribute not only to our understanding of the dying process but to our care of terminally-ill patients, our ability to help grieving families, and our approach to suicidal patients" (p. 1193). Integrating the Near-Death Experience into the curriculum will expand the nurse's knowledge of the dying process.

REFERENCES

Bush, N. (1983). "The near-death experience in children: Shades of the prison-house reopening." *Anabiosis, 3,* 177-193.

Flynn, C. (1982). "Meanings and implications of NDE transformations: Some preliminary findings and implications." *Anabiosis, 2,* 3-15.

Green, J. and Friedman, P. (1983). "Near-death experiences in a Southern California population." *Anabiosis, 3,* 77-96.

Greyson, B. (1983). "The near-death experience scale: Construction, reliability and validity." *Journal of Nervous and Mental Disease, 171,* 369-375.

Greyson, B. and Stevenson, I. (1980). "The phenomenology of near-death experiences." *American Journal of Psychiatry, 137,* 1193-1196.

Hinton, J. (1963). "The physical and mental distress of the dying." *Quarterly Journal of Medicine, 32,* 1-21.

International Association for Near-Death Studies, Box U-20, The University of Connecticut, 06268.

Kastenbaum, R. (1979). *Between Life and Death*. New York: Springer Pub. Co.

Moody, R. (1975). *Life After Life*. New York: Bantam Books.

Osis, K. (1961). *Deathbed Observations by Physicians and Nurses*. New York: Parapsychology Foundation.

Osis, K. and Heraldsson, E. (1977). *At the Hour of Death*. New York: Avon Books.

Ring, K. (1981). "Paranormal and other non-ordinary aspects of near-death experiences: Implications of a new paradigm." *Essence*, 5, 33-51.

Ring, K. (1980). *Life at Death: A Scientific Investigation of the Near-death Experience*. New York: Coward, McCann & Geoghegan.

Sabom, M. (1982). *Recollections of Death: A Medical Investigation*. New York: Harper & Row.

Schneidman, E. (1976). *Death: Current Perspectives*. California: Mayfield.

Guidelines for Death Education as a Developmental Process

Mary A. Seidel

As professionals concerned with educating students about the process of death and the care of the dying person and his or her family, we face a constant challenge. This challenge involves the continuing struggle to incorporate "sufficient" time and content about a specific area of clinical practice into the ever-crowded curricula programs of nursing, medicine and other health fields. This paper, using the nursing profession as an example, proposes some guidelines that can be used to assist educators in developing an overall program in death education for professionals in their own respective fields.

Four steps have been included in developing these guidelines for death education; (1) the identification of the basic knowledge and skills in the area of thanatology necessary for practitioners, (2) the recognition that these skills will be learned as the student develops professionally, (3) the establishment of a time line for the teaching and supervision of such knowledge and skills throughout the person's career, and (4) the exploration of ways to incorporate this knowledge and skill development into (a) the formal curricula of professional programs, (b) semi-formal training opportunities such as workshops and continuing education programs, and (c) ongoing informal processes of role modeling and support groups.

DEATH EDUCATION AS A CONTINUING PROCESS

Education about death may be defined as "a developmental process that transmits to people and society valid death-related knowledge and its implications for subsequent change in attitudes and behavior" (Leviton 1977, p. 44). Due to its social and psychological consequences, death education should be introduced in a developmental and systematic manner. Learning about death and dying should be considered a continuous process that cannot be achieved after one course, at one workshop, or in writing one paper.

Many factors influence professionals as they learn about death and dying, and they should be considered in planning educational programs. Some include: (1) the clinical setting, (2) the role of the professional, (3) personal characteristics of the individual, and (4) the level of clinical practice. This paper will focus on the influence of the level of clinical practice in guiding programs on death education. However, a brief mention of the other influences is warranted.

First, death experiences vary with the settings in which professionals work, for the nature of, and contact with, death is vastly different in community health, hospice care, and critical care units. Deaths may be anticipated events or unexpected emergencies, which occur frequently or seldom. These factors clearly affect an individual's skills, feelings, and attitudes. Second, the role that professionals play in a particular setting also influences what they need to know and what aspects of death education would be most relevant. For example, a head nurse or chief resident might need additional measures that help in directing and supporting other staff. Third, the personal characteristics of the individual professional, such as educational level, age, religious affiliation, and ethnic origin (Gaston 1980; Kalish and Reynolds 1977), play an important part in influencing perceptions of death and dying. These characteristics contribute to how individuals "see their world" and subsequently, their professional role. Personal beliefs or experiences may enhance or hinder professional responsibilities; therefore, it is important to understand and appreciate the relationship between these two aspects in a professional's life (Seidel 1981).

DEVELOPMENT OF CLINICAL PRACTICE

The final influence identified involves the level of clinical practice—a major focus of this paper, as it affects planning programs for death education. Benner's work, *From Novice to Expert* (1984), suggests that the complexity and responsibility of nursing practice today require long-term, ongoing career development. Benner systematically observed and interviewed different nurses from various settings, using the Dreyfus Model of Skill Acquisition (Dreyfus 1980). This model suggests that an individual passes through five levels in the acquisition and development of a skill: novice, advanced beginner, competent, proficient, and expert. With the strong belief that death education is also a developmental process, I suggest that educators use these levels of practice skill to plan and implement ongoing educational experiences that will promote quality care for dying persons and their families.

For decades medicine has promoted a step-wise transition in clinical practice with its well-recognized, though admittedly not perfect, residency programs. Nursing, on the other hand, has expected a nurse to "function" as an RN the day he or she receives the state license. We have not identified or accepted the realities of developing clinical skill and expertise. Until now!

In understanding the differences between the experienced nurse and the novice, educators can tailor specific programs about death and plan learning experiences with the dying person and the family for each level. Nurses at the NOVICE level (I) are the beginners with no experience in the many situations they encounter in the clinical setting. (The professional nursing student is included in this category.) These individuals are expected to perform certain tasks. They are taught in terms of objective attributes which are features of the task that can be recognized without situational experience. Common attributes include: weight, intake and output, vital signs, and other such objective, measurable parameters of the patient's condition. They are taught rules to guide action with respect to these different attributes, such as how to assess fluid balance. Novices frequently are unable to use discretionary judgment. Because they lack experience, they must use context-free rules to guide their performance. Unfortunately, no rules can tell a novice which tasks are most relevant in a real situation or when an exception to the rule is in order. It is amazing and somewhat disturbing to consider the numbers of nurses in this first level of practice whom we find in the hospital setting, working under stressful conditions with little or no supervision.

Nurses at the ADVANCED BEGINNER level (II) are those who

can demonstrate marginally acceptable performance, those who have coped with enough real situations to note the recurrent, meaningful, situational components, called aspects. According to the Dreyfus Model, "aspects" mean overall, global characteristics that require prior experience in actual situations for recognition. One example is assessing a patient's readiness to learn. Aspect recognition is dependent on prior experience. These nurses can draw from previous experience with patients in similar situations. Instructors or preceptors can provide guidelines for recognizing these aspects, but these guidelines are dependent on knowing what the aspects sound like and look like in a patient care situation.

The advanced beginner or instructor for these nurses can formulate guidelines for actions which integrate as many attributes and aspects as possible. However, these guidelines tend to ignore their differential importance. All aspects are treated alike and are equally important. The novice and advanced beginner in strange and new situations must concentrate on remembering the rules they've been taught. Aspect recognition, like the ability to discriminate various breath sounds, is an important goal at this level. At the next level of practice, the nurse will focus on the more advanced clinical skill of judging the relative importance of differential aspects of the situation. Advanced beginners need support in the clinical unit in setting priorities, since they are only beginning to perceive recurrent, meaningful patterns in their clinical practice.

Nurses at the COMPETENT level (III) have been "on the job" for several years. They begin to see their actions in terms of long-range goals or plans and they are consciously aware of these plans. These dictate to them which attributes and aspects of the current and contemplated future situations are considered most important and which can be ignored. Competent nurses develop a perspective based on considerable conscious, abstract, and analytic study of the problem. The competency stage is characterized by a feeling of mastery and the ability to cope with and manage the many contingencies of clinical nursing. While these nurses lack the speed and flexibility of the nurse at the next stage, their deliberate planning helps achieve a level of efficiency and organization in their practice.

Many nurses stay at this level, which is supported and reinforced by the institution and perceived as ideal by their supervisors. Standard and routine procedures enable them to manage the high turnover of patients found in many clinical settings.

Nurses at the PROFICIENT level (IV) develop with continued practice. They perceive situations as wholes, rather than in terms of aspects. Their performance is guided by maxims. Experience teaches these nurses what typical events to expect, how to modify plans, and how to recognize the normal. The holistic understanding of the proficient nurse improves their decision making and makes it less laborious by considering fewer options and honing in on an accurate region of the problem. A deep understanding of the situation, including the subtle nuances, provides these nurses with a sense of what is important to take into consideration and what should be ignored (for example, how to wean a patient from a respirator).

Nurses at the final EXPERT level (V) no longer rely on analytical principles (such as rules, guidelines, and maxims) but demonstrate an intuitive grasp of the situation and zero in on the accurate region of the problem without wasteful consideration of long-range or possible problem situations. They operate from a deep understanding of the situation that is frustrating to capture in verbal descriptions of their performance. Their knowledge of goals and possible outcomes can be helpful in expanding the scope of practice of nurses who are less proficient.

A vision of what is possible separates competent performance from proficient or expert performance. This vision can raise the sights of the competent nurse and facilitate movement to the proficient stage. Expert nurses must be encouraged to describe and share the examples of interventions that "made a difference," and to expose others to their processing of clinical situations and their highly skilled analytical ability. In this way some of the knowledge embedded in the expert's practice becomes visible.

PLANNING EDUCATIONAL PROGRAMS

With these five levels in mind, we can now consider how to incorporate the necessary knowledge and skill development in the formal curricula, semiformal training opportunities, and ongoing informal socialization processes for professionals.

Nursing baccalaureate programs must provide students with the basic knowledge and skills that can be applied in many situations of patient care. Often, care for the dying is either consciously or unconsciously avoided. Some schools choose to integrate concepts of death and dying into their curricula, but often this thread is lost and limited to an occasional lecture in one or two courses.

It is very important that, along with the basic skill acquisition to perform necessary tasks associated with patient care, students learn basic communication and assessment skills that will assist them in working in more complex situations with dying persons and families. They must learn about the process of dying and stages of grieving and have an opportunity to explore their own attitudes, beliefs and feelings. This learning can, of course, be best organized in a specific course on death and dying which can be offered as a required or an elective advanced clinical opportunity.

All nursing students deserve the opportunity to work with a dying patient and his or her family at least once during the nursing program so that they can receive necessary support, supervision and guidance from clinical faculty and staff. Too often the recent graduate must face the first professional encounter with death alone and without support and supervision. Since nurses at this level lack the skills to use discretionary judgment so necessary in working with the dying person, a faculty member or staff person should work with the student at all times so that he/she can learn from the more experienced nurse. Clinical seminars can also be a useful avenue to explore problems and feelings about these clinical situations.

The new graduate in a staff position needs much of the same support and guidance as the student. A good orientation program in clinical settings should include opportunity to learn about emergency care and code procedures along with a chance to practice such skills. New programs using preceptors (more experienced staff) are excellent ways to support new staff in working with difficult and more complex clinical situations.

Advanced Beginners (II), in their first months of practice, need the continued staff support that the new graduate needs. Even after extended orientation programs, young or relatively new nurses are too often expected to perform with speed and ease. These individuals would do well working with a preceptor to discuss care of the dying patients and their families, for this may be the first time that they have full responsibility in such clinical situations. Assuming that their basic skills are honed, and feeling more secure that they won't do anything wrong or "dumb" or embarrassing in this emotionally difficult situation, these nurses, with proper supervision and support, can focus on improving their communication skills and their ability to set priorities in delivering care.

Nursing rounds by more advanced nurses on specific units would be helpful to discuss specific patients who are dying. Inservice programs by experts in the field of thanatology from the hospital or nearby university faculty can also serve as a useful learning and support function.

Nurses at the Competent level (III) have several years' experience and are now feeling a mastery and ability to cope with and manage the demands of the clinical setting. Their ability to plan and organize can assist less experienced nurses. But they too need the continued support from more experienced professionals to improve the quality of their care. Nurses at this stage seem to benefit from experience in decision-making games and simulations that give them practice in planning for and coordinating multiple, complex, patient care demands. They can focus on the subtleties of working in tense situations, on meeting the varying and sometimes opposite needs of the dying person and his or her family, and on how to coordinate and communicate with the other members of the health team. Until this stage, nurses are usually not ready to function in this role.

At this time, many nurses choose to go back to school for specialized preparation at the master's level, or to begin to take some courses, attend workshops or continuing educational programs. They are ready to learn more, and they usually have a good idea about what they want to study. Graduate courses, inservice programs, and workshops on more advanced concepts about death and dying, such as ethical issues and home care issues, should be offered on a regular basis by hospitals, universities and colleges, and professional organizations.

Nurses at the PROFICIENT level (IV), with continued practice, demonstrate a holistic understanding of the clinical situations they encounter. They should be tapped for their knowledge and skills to work with other staff on the clinical unit because of their ability to recognize whole situations. Few nurses at this level of practice are found in clinical settings. Too often they move to other positions in or out of the hospital setting. Clinical staff positions have not been reinforcing enough to keep proficient nurses. Now, with clinical ladder programs, nurses with advanced clinical expertise can be recognized and rewarded. Nurses at the proficient level should be recruited and valued for the quality of care they provide dying patients and their families. As such, they serve as significant role models for other staff members.

Few courses or inservice programs are geared to nurses at this level. Offering context-free principles and rules will leave proficient nurses frustrated. Proficient performers are best taught by the use of case studies where their ability to grasp the situation is solicited and taxed. Experts from a community or regional level should be invited to come to clinical settings for conferences and discussions of such case studies. Nurses should also be given educational leave to attend special courses and travel opportunities to participate in conferences at the regional or national level to advance and expand their own knowledge and skills. On a day-to-day basis, proficient nurses can benefit from support groups either within the hospital setting or on a regional or community level.

Nurses at the EXPERT level (V), with their extensive experience, have an intuitive grasp of the situation and can focus on the particular problem at hand without unnecessary processing. Their deep understanding of situations can contribute a tremendous amount of valuable insight for improving the care of the dying patient and family. Mechanisms should be set up in hospital situations where expert nurses can share their successful interventions with patients, families and staff. Their knowledge of goals and possible outcomes can be useful in expanding the scope of nursing practice. By encouraging the expert to describe clinical situations where his or her intervention made a difference, some of the knowledge embedded in the expert's practice becomes visible. Not only does this give nurses the opportunity to reinforce the skills at this level of practice but it also helps educators to identify what is needed in preparing practitioners to give quality care to dying patients and families.

CONCLUSION

This paper used Benner's application of the Dreyfus Model of Skill Acquisition to create guidelines for death education as a developmental process. Using examples from the nursing profession, the intent has been to present clearly the five developmental stages individuals pass through from novice to expert.

The Dreyfus Model of Skill Acquisition (1980) incorporates the value of experience into the educational process. Experience, as understood and used in the acquisition of expertise, is not the mere passage of time. Experience is the refinement of preconceived notions and theory by encountering many actual practical situations that add nuances or shades of differences to theory (Benner 1982).

In summary, educators and practitioners can facilitate death education as a developmental process by providing a variety of courses, learning opportunities, and support systems for health care professionals at each level of practice. The planning and implementation of these programs are a joint responsibility of educational institutions and service agencies in their mutual goal of improving the quality of care given to dying persons and their families.

REFERENCES

Benner, P. (1984). *From Novice to Expert*. Menlo Park: Addison-Wesley Publishing Company.

———. (1982). "From novice to expert." *American Journal of Nursing*, *82*(3), 402-407.

Dreyfus, S. and Dreyfus, H. (1980). "A five stage model of the mental activities involved in directed skill acquisition." Supported by the U.S. Air Force, Office of Scientific Research (AFSC) under contract F49620-C-0063 with the University of California-Berkeley, February, 1980. (Unpublished study).

Gaston, S. K. (1980). "Death and midlife crisis." *Journal of Psychiatric Nursing and Mental Health Services*, *18*, 31-35.

Kalish, R. A. and Reynolds, D. K. (1977). "The role of age in death attitudes." *Death Education*, *1*(2), 205-230.

Leviton, D. (1977). "The scope of death education." *Death Education*, *1*(1), 44.

Seidel, M. A. (1981). "Death education: A continuing process for nurses." *Topics in Clinical Nursing*, *3*(3), 87-97.

ADDITIONAL READING

Martin, L. and Collier, P. (1975). "Attitudes toward death: Survey of nursing students." *Journal of Nursing Education, 14*(1), 28-35.
Wise, D. (1974). "Learning about dying." *Nursing Outlook, 22*(1), 42-44.

The Value of Computer-Assisted Instruction in Death Education

Madeline E. Lambrecht

Computer technology is causing multifarious changes in today's society. According to Billings (1984), social values influence educational practice, hence educators need to be particularly sensitive to computer applications when developing teaching and learning strategies. This premise has special relevance for death educators in terms of innovative instructional planning for the future.

Current instructional applications of computers in health care include: (a) drill and practice programs, (b) tutorial programs, (c) gaming programs, (d) simulations, and (e) computerized test banks. Most of these applications are underutilized in the field of death education and virtually none address the issue of awareness related to one's own death and dying in more than a superficial manner.

A review of the recent literature supports a need for awareness related to one's own death and dying as a prerequisite for future effective practice. Backer, Hannon and Russel (1982) cited self-awareness in relation to death and dying as a significant issue in the nursing profession. According to Lowenberg (1976), nurses use so much energy to handle their own feelings about death that they may be unable to recognize or deal with their clients' needs. Death education with emphasis upon self-awareness was utilized as a resource to alleviate this problem. Other professionals, including Simpson (1979), stress the importance of attitudinal objectives as well as cognitive goals in developing effective death education programs.

In recognition of the need for self-awareness related to death and dying and the unique interactive capabilities of the computer, Lambrecht (1982, 1983) developed a PLATO (Programmed Logic for Automatic Teaching Operations) lesson to help students achieve effective objectives in the personalization of the death experience.

The lesson is entitled "Death: A Personal Encounter" (Copyright 1981 by the University of Delaware), and is programmed to run on the PLATO system. The rationale for choosing a computer as a teaching/learning strategy to facilitate awareness related to one's own death was based on four issues: (a) personalization of instruction, (b) branching capabilities, (c) immediacy of feedback, and (d) anonymity. Personalization of instruction is achieved through initial data supplied by the student. The computer's memory recalls specific information and presents it at appropriate times in the lesson. Branching capabilities allow the student to explore personally meaningful avenues of inquiry, yet the computer reminds the student that other areas of concern might also be explored. The interactive features of the computer allow for immediate feedback for some of the student's concerns and fears. Lastly, the computer provides anonymity for the initial exploration of one's feelings about death and dying.

The lession is considered a *first step* in the development of self-awareness related to death and dying. The lesson contains no didactic material. Rather it is entirely focused on the elicitation of feelings and beliefs related to death in general and to one's own death in particular. According to Lambrecht (1981), the following are the lesson objectives:

- to think about death consciously;
- to identify personal attitudes, beliefs, and values relevant to death and dying;
- to describe your feelings about your own death;
- to recognize that anxiety concerning death is often a reflection of personal fears related to your own death.

The lesson consists of two parts: (1) an assessment of personal attitudes and beliefs related to death and dying, and (2) a simulation in which the student contracts a terminal illness and is actively engaged (if she/he so chooses) in the decision-making process from the choice of medical treatment (or nontreatment) to preferred death rituals. The simulation incorporates personal data generated in the first part of the lesson to further intensify the personalization aspect of the death experience. Components of the lesson include several self-assessments of anxiety level related to progression through the lesson, personalized graphics such as a tombstone with the student's name and date of death, a nearly factual death certificate, burial arrangements, and lastly, a written eulogy for one's self.

Numerous precautions are taken throughout the lesson in recognition of the highly sensitive nature of the subject matter. Recent experience with terminal illness and/or death is assessed early in the lesson and the student always has the option to leave the lesson at any point. A resource guide is provided as part of the lesson itself.

The lesson has been utilized in both the undergraduate and graduate departments of nursing at the University of Delaware over a period of four years. Response to the lesson documented by an on-line questionnaire has been very positive. Information generated throughout the lesson is saved in a student data file which provides useful data for lesson revision and research efforts. These outcomes indicate that further exploration of computer-assisted instruction in death education has considerable merit.

REFERENCES

Backer, B.A., Hannon, N., & Russel, N.A. (1982). Death and Dying – Individuals and Institutions. New York: John Wiley & Sons.

Billings, D.M. (1984). "Evaluating computer-assisted instruction." *Nursing Outlook, 32* (1), 50-53.

Lambrecht, M.E. (1981). Death: A personal encounter (Computer program). Newark, DE: University of Delaware (PLATO system).

Lambrecht, M.E. (1982). PLATO as a teaching device in death education. *About Teaching* (no. 13). Newark, DE: University of Delaware, Center for Teaching Effectiveness.

Lambrecht, M.E. (1983). PLATO helps nursing students confront their unexpressed feelings about death and dying. *Proceedings of the Ninth International Conference on Improving University Teaching*, (pp. 330-338). Dublin, Ireland: The University of Maryland University College and National Institute for Higher Education, Dublin.

Lowenberg, J.S. (1976). Working through feelings about death. In A.M. Earle, N.T. Argondizzo, & A.H. Kutscher (Eds.), *The Nurse as Caregiver for the Terminal Patient and His Family*, (pp. 125-127). New York: Columbia University Press.

Simpson, M.A. (1979). Death education – where is thy sting? *Death Education, 3*, 165-173.

A Study of the Relationship Between Knowledge and Attitudes of Nurses in Practice Related to the Near-Death Experience

Evelyn R. Hayes
Roberta M. Orne

Approximately 40% of people who survive clinical death or a near-fatal encounter with death report some variant of a phenomenon known as the near-death experience (NDE). Gallup (1982) reports that approximately eight million people in this country alone have experienced this phenomenon. A near-death experience most commonly occurs when an individual comes close to death in an accident, a suicide attempt, or during an operation.

Basing their reports on thousands of detailed descriptions of the phenomenon, researchers have identified components of the NDE which appear to unfold in a characteristic way. Ring (1980) has labeled his classic five-stage sequential model the "core near-death experience." Most people do not experience all five stages. The latter stages are less commonly or never encountered.

Ring describes Stage I as the affective accompaniment of the experience and estimates that approximately 60% of the people in his study report this aspect. Survivors report feelings of absolute peace, contentment, and well-being in this stage. Individuals often say that there is just "no way" to describe it.

Individuals who experience Stage II, approximately 45% of Ring's sample, speak of a sense of separation from one's physical body. Typically, individuals report looking down on their bodies, with a feeling of natural detachment, as if they were spectators.

Ring has labeled the third stage "entering the darkness," and it seems to represent a transitional phase. Those encountering this phase describe moving (floating or drifting) through a nondimensional tunnel or dark space. Approximately 25% of Ring's study subjects experienced this "peaceful blackness," and some describe movement from this darkness toward a brilliant golden or white engulfing light.

Stage IV, or "seeing the light," has been reported by approximately 20% of people who experienced NDE. The light is further described as warm, restful and comfortable.

"Entering the light," the final stage, is the least commonly encountered. About 10% report this. Those who experience it speak of entering another world or setting often described as a paradise of indescribable, wondrous beauty and color. At this stage, some report encountering deceased loved ones while others become aware of a "felt presence" often recounted as God-like. Often a life review occurs during this stage, but that may occur in other phases as well.

Both immediate and ongoing reactions to an NDE are said to vary considerably from person to person. It has been reported that some individuals have no immediate reaction to the NDE. Most individuals, however, have profound and often mixed affective responses over time. These may include euphoria, anger, relief, agitation, sadness, depression, peace, and contentment. Furthermore, recent studies document drastic changes in a patient's life style and attitudes in the months and years following a near-death experience (Ring, 1980).

While the near-death experience has been recorded in the literature since ancient times, little research addressed this issue, with the exception of 19th century physical research, until the mid-1970s. The work of Dr. Elizabeth Kübler-Ross (1975) and Dr. Raymond Moody (1975, 1977) stimulated a great deal of interest within the scientific and lay communities. There are now literally scores of scholars and researchers involved in near-death studies throughout the world (Greyson 1981; Gallop 1982; Gabbard and Twenlow 1981; Lundahl 1981; Noyes 1979; Osis and Haraldsson 1977 a and b; Rodin 1980; Sabom 1982; and Sabom and Kreutziger 1978). As a result, there is greater acceptance of such reports within the medical and scientific communities. Skepticism, however, remains regarding the interpretation and meaning of the experience. Growing interest and research have generally broadened awareness of the NDE as a psychological phenomenon and increased knowledge about the event itself and the lives of those who experience it.

REVIEW OF THE LITERATURE

Studies indicate that a person's reluctance to initiate discussions or share the event is often due to an assumption that no one would believe him or her, neither family nor close friends (Sabom 1982; Oakes 1981). Sabom reports that many patients privately question their sanity and wish to be reassured that the NDE is not evidence of mental illness. It is not uncommon to find survivors suppressing their near-death experiences for five, ten, twenty years or more. It should not be surprising, then, that for many the experience remains unsettling and unresolved.

On the other hand, some individuals do share their experiences — more readily when the health care provider is perceived as believeing the accounts and respectful of their feelings (Oakes 1981). In fact, a trusted care giver is often asked to be with a patient when significant others are first told about the NDE. A trusted nurse more often hears NDE accounts than do other health professionals.

Yet the nursing literature contains little reference to the NDE, little detail about the nature of the phenomenon or the tremendous impact it seems to have on patients and loved ones, and few guidelines for appropriate, effective nursing care. Only two studies with small samples have examined nurses' attitudes toward the NDE and its relationship to client care.

NEED FOR THE STUDY

While the data are limited, they do suggest that the perceptions of those who experience NDE and their ability to solve problems and to cope are significantly influenced by professional providers, often positively by nurses. Little is known, however, about the basis on which nurses plan and evaluate care for these patients and their loved ones. Specifically, no study has been done to determine the extent of nurses' knowledge about the NDE and only limited data exist about nurses' attitudes.

With increasingly sophisticated technology and resuscitative measures, the number of individuals surviving near-death episodes is growing and with it the frequency of NDE reports. This heightens the possibility the nurse will encounter these patients in practice. A study would be especially timely because the near-death experience phenomenon has only recently been acknowledged as a psychological phenomenon and it is not included in the course content and experiential learnings of most basic and graduate nursing programs.

CONCEPTUAL FRAMEWORK

According to the crisis theory conceptual model of nursing practice, the study framework, individuals are constantly faced with a need to solve problems in order to maintain dynamic equilibrium. Crisis theorists (Caplan 1964; Aguilera & Messick 1974) have emphasized that the kind of support an individual receives, especially one under increased stress, is vital to resolution of the event.

Inherent in the crisis model of nursing practice is the construct that knowledge and attitudes influence perceptions.

It is suggested that when the nurse's repertoire of knowledge is limited or inaccurate, negative or ambivalent attitudes may be held and, in turn, they may influence the response to the patient and family. It may be further speculated that distorted patient perceptions could be reinforced or neglected, collaborative problem solving avoided or thwarted, and patient/family coping compromised and/or problematic. Conversely, if the nurse's knowledge is broad based and accurate, a more positive attitude is likely. It may be speculated, then, that this allows the nurse greater comprehension of the situation and a better ability to clarify perceptions, encourage collaborative problem solving, and provide support for patient/family coping with activation of the growth potential as a primary goal.

PURPOSE

The purpose of this descriptive correlational study was to elicit data regarding nurses' knowledge and attitudes about the NDE. Study findings were projected to comprise a significant base line of initial nursing data from which direction for further study and implication for practice might be derived.

The research questions generated were:

1. What is the extent of perceived and "actual" knowledge of the NDE among nurses in practice?
2. What attitudes currently prevail with respect to NDE among nurses in practice?
3. What are the sources of that knowledge?
4. What is the range of nursing intervention nurses identify as appropriate for the NDE patient?
5. What is the relationship between nurses' knowledge and attitudes toward NDE?

METHODOLOGY

A convenience sample of 1600 was drawn from registered nurses, employed full or part time, in six acute care and two community health care settings in Connecticut, New York and Massachusetts. All nurses in each agency were asked to participate voluntarily and anonymously by independently completing a questionnaire. Nine hundred twelve nurses returned completed questionnaires for a return rate of 61%.

Of the 912 participating nurses, 97% were female. Approximately half were less than 29 years old, while approximately 7% of the sample were fifty or older.

Forty-one percent of the subjects held a baccalaureate degree, 34% a diploma, 14% an associate degree and the remaining 11% a master's degree or higher. Fifty percent of these nurses had earned their degrees in the last five years while it had been fifteen years or more for 19% of the sample.

Using a self-administered, investigator-developed questionnaire, respondents self-selected into two groups based on their perception of knowledge of the near-death experience. The instrument, with accompanying cover letter, took 10 to 20 minutes to complete, and was composed of three color-coded parts:

A. *Demographic data on respondents.* The last question, "Are you familiar with the phenomenon of NDE?" determined which section of the instrument the respondent would complete.

B. *Responses from nurses familiar with NDE.* Of this group of nurses, we asked questions regarding perception of knowledge, measured extent of knowledge, elicited attitudes about NDE and identified appropriate nursing interventions. This section had 20 items.

C. *Responses from nurses not familiar with or not sure about NDE.* This group of nurses was directed to read a scenario of the NDE and then respond to questions about attitude and indicate interventions such a patient might need. Appropriate interventions were those judged to be supportive by at least two persons knowledgeable about NDE. This section had eight items. Thus, respondents completed parts A and B or parts A and C.

The instrument had content validity in that persons knowledgeable about NDE provided input at every stage in its development. Test-retest reliability conducted with 30 graduate nursing students was 0.91, which was deemed to be satisfactory.

RESULTS

Within the acute care agencies, the vast majority of nurses practiced in eleven major specialty units. The largest number of nurses sampled (29%) were employed on medical and surgical units, and 25% were employed in intensive care units, the emergency room, the operating and recovery rooms. The remaining 46% practiced in community health, oncology, maternity, pediatric, psychiatry, and rehabilitation units and a variety of other areas including nursing service.

Forty-one percent in the overall sample had experienced the death of a significant other within the last two years. Overall, 57% of the sample was Catholic, 30% Protestant, 6.8% Jewish, and 6% had no religious preference. In addition, when asked to what extent subjects were guided by their religious precepts, 9% replied "not at all," 5% "a great deal," while the majority were evenly distributed between the extremes on a 6-point Likert Scale.

Familiarity with the NDE based on the individual's perceptions was queried. Seventy percent of the respondents indicated familiarity, 10% indicated they were not familiar with it and 20% were not sure if they were familiar with the NDE phenomenon.

The 70% who indicated familiarity with NDE were asked to indicate their perception of the extent of this knowledge on a 6-point Likert Scale from very limited to very extensive. The findings were distributed along a bell-shaped curve with 55% in the two central categories. Those who perceived more limited knowledge accounted for 30% and those who perceived more extensive knowledge accounted for 15%.

A total "actual" knowledge score was calculated for each participant. These scores ranged from 1 to 16. Sixteen was the highest possible score. Ten percent of the respondents scored 9 or above. Hence, 90% had scores of 50% or less on the total "actual" knowledge score.

Participants' responses to an open-ended question indicating their attitude toward the NDE fell into the following categories: curiosity = 426 (50.1%); belief = 312 (36.7%); spiritual = 27 (3.2%); disbelief = 26 (3.1%); physiological = 6 (0.7%); and other = 53 (62%).

When asked for their interpretation of an NDE, 41% felt it was spiritual in nature, 12% said it was a physiological response, 7% interpreted it as a psychic experience and 31% said they simply didn't have any idea.

Several sources of knowledge for the NDE were identified. Forty percent indicated that the lay media, including television, radio, newspapers, and magazines, were their predominant sources of this knowledge. The second most frequently cited source was patients and patients' relatives; this was followed by nursing education, professional journal or text, other, and colleague.

Respondents were asked to list interventions they would use specifically with NDE clients. These were categorized into six major responses. Eighty-six percent of nurses listed "encourage discussion or listen," 69% stated they would "offer support and empathy," 39% felt it important to intervene by "referring to and providing more information to the patient," 12% said it was important to "gather more data," while 4% included "research" in their list of planned interventions.

To address the last research question, a Pearson Product Moment Correlation was calculated between total "actual" knowledge score and current attitude. This correlation was .2205, which is low but significant beyond .001.

NURSING IMPLICATIONS AND CONCLUSION

While further research will require a more comprehensive and precise instrument to measure nurses' knowledge and attitudes prior to increasing sample size and comparing geographic, interdisciplinary and cross cultural differences, the present findings have significant relevance for nursing education and practice.

The perceived NDE knowledge of the nurses was not validated by the actual knowledge scores. Professional nursing and allied health texts and journals, however, are virtually devoid of reference to the NDE. It was not a surprising finding of the study that the primary source of NDE information was the lay press and media. While some lay reports are accurate and informative, others distort facts, promote misinformation, and sensationalize the NDE. This poses a challenge to the nurse educator.

It is important that the study found that 96% of the sample did not feel adequately informed about the phenomenon and its implications for practice and wished to learn more. Data from this study will facilitate the design and implementation of NDE educational programs designed to meet the needs of nurses and students.

During the course of the data analysis, it became evident that nurses were keenly interested in this emerging dimension of professional practice. In addition to completing the questionnaire, many subjects used the tool as a vehicle to describe personal and patient NDE accounts. They wrote at length about the dilemmas they experienced and the dilemmas expressed by a patient or a patient's family members.

A variety of appropriate interventions for NDE patients was identified. These behaviors need to be explored further before recommendations are made.

Studies in related sociological fields indicate that increased knowledge correlates with positive attitudes. Therefore, it was not surprising to find a direct relationship between nurses' knowledge and attitude toward the NDE.

Overall study findings are significant for nursing practice, education, and research by constituting a data base for future studies, formulating hypotheses to be tested in future research, and promoting direction for the design of NDE educational programs for nurses.

REFERENCES

Aguilera, D. and Messick, J. (1974). *Crisis Intervention: Theory and Methodology*. St. Louis: C.V. Mosby.

Caplan, G. (1964). *Principles of Preventive Psychiatry*. New York: Basic Books Inc.

Gabbard, C. and Twenlow, S. (1981). "Explanatory hypotheses for near-death experiences." *Revision, 4*, 68-71.

Gallup, C. (1982). *Adventures in Immortality*. New York: McGraw-Hill.

Greyson, B. (1981). "Near-death experiences and attempted suicide." *Suicide and Life-threatening Behavior, 11*, 10-16.

Kübler-Ross, E. (1975). *Death: The Final Stages of Growth*. Englewood Cliffs, NJ: Prentice-Hall.

Lundahl, C. (1981). "Directions in near-death research." *Death Education, 5*, 135-142.

Moody, R. (1975). *Life After Life*. Atlanta: Mockingbird Books.

Moody, R. (1977). *Reflections of Life After Life*. Atlanta: Mockingbird Books.

Noyes, R. (1979). "Near-death experiences: Their interpretation and significance." In R. Kastenbaum (Ed.). *Between Life and Death*. 73-87. New York: Springer.

Oakes, A. (1981). "Near-death events and critical care nursing." *Topics in Clinical Nursing, 3*, 61-78.

Osis, K. and Haraldsson, E. (1977a). *At the Hour of Death*. New York: Avon Books.

Osis, K. and Haraldsson, E. (1977b). "Deathbed observations by physicians and nurses: A cross-cultural survey." *Journal of the American Society for Psychical Research, 71*, 237-259.

Ring, K. (1980). *Life at Death; A Scientific Investigation of the Near-death Experience*. New York: Coward, McCann and Geoghegan.

Rodin, E. (1980). "The reality of death experiences, a personal perspective." *Journal of Nervous and Mental Disease*, *168*(5), 259-260.

Sabom, M. and Kreutziger, S. (1978). "Physicians evaluate the near-death experience." *Theta*, *6*(4), 1-6.

Sabom, M. (1982). *Recollections of Death: A Medical Investigation*. New York: Harper and Row.

ADDITIONAL READING

Infante, M. S. (Ed.) (1982). *Crisis Theory: A Framework for Nursing Practice*. Reston, VA: Reston Publishing Co.

Oakes, A. (1978). "The Lazarus syndrome: Caring for patients who've returned from the dead." *Registered Nurse*, *41*(6), 54-57.

Osis, K. (1961). *Deathbed Observations by Physicians and Nurses*. New York: Parapsychology Foundation.

Ring, K. (1982). *Near-death Studies: A New Area of Consciousness Research*. Storrs, CT: International Association for Near-death Studies.

SECTION II:
COPING APPROACHES AND THE THANATOLOGY CURRICULUM

Grieving:
An Essential Topic
in Allied Health Education

Lucy G. Bruce
D. Lisa Leonard
John G. Bruhn

Grief is an inevitable and recurring aspect of human life. Grief, itself, is a process. It is part of normal growth and development, yet it is often overlooked or excluded from the human growth and development courses taught to health professionals (Simon 1971), although such courses are becoming more common.

A recent survey reported that 50% of medical schools and 45% of nursing schools offer at least one course on the topic of death and dying (Sinacore 1981). And several programs to teach the subject have been described (Dietrich 1980; Harris 1980; Dickens & Mullen 1983; Purtilo 1972; Lutticken et al. 1974; Gammage et al. 1976; and Bridle 1977).

Physicians may be involved in assisting the patient to cope with grief, but other health professionals will be a part of the process.

81

They may be the patients' only source of information about their progress and hopes for recovery. Patients grieve in different ways and the ways in which they cope with grief can affect their progress in therapy. Health professionals must have some insight into their own grief experiences in order to assist those patients and their families who are grieving (Miller 1977). Helping the patient with adaptation to loss is part of treatment and rehabilitation (Bruhn 1981; Zelinsky & Thorson 1983; Goldstein 1977; and Stewart & Rossier 1978).

CONCEPT OF GRIEF: A DEVELOPMENTAL PERSPECTIVE

Grief is usually thought of in terms of death or separation from a family member, relative, or friend, but it may occur with any type of loss — loss of a job, perceived loss of status, or even loss of a prized possession. It is a part of the experience in a change in physical or mental health, especially if surgery or institutionalization is required or the diagnosis involves chronic illness, disability, or terminal illness.

Grief is a life experience that is not restricted to any one age group, although the meaning of grief and how an individual copes with it is best understood in terms of age or stage of development. There are limitations in categorizing the life cycle into time periods or levels of development but some markers are needed to monitor an individual's progress. Development is orderly, not random. Different types of development are important at different times; some periods are more significant than others in development periods during which a life event has its greatest impact. There are wide ranges in normal development, and differences among individuals may be understood in terms of the normal range (Kaluger & Kaluger 1984).

An individual's grief is influenced by the interrelationships between the completion of past and present developmental tasks. Successful development depends upon accomplishment of tasks at each stage. Failure with these tasks at any stage affects the ability to succeed with future tasks and results in unhappiness and societal disapproval (Havighurst 1979). An individual's experience with grief is cumulative, and the way the individual copes with each new grief experience is influenced by previous experiences and by the degree to which they were satisfactorily resolved.

The developmental tasks in adolescence and middle adulthood stand in sharp contrast to one another (see Table 1). The adolescent tasks are both present and future oriented, with completion or accomplishment at a later time. Adolescents must achieve emotional independence and learn to make and accept the consequences of choices. Middle-aged adults are predominantly present-oriented with one important task, assisting teenage children to become responsible and happy adults. In order to do so, they rely heavily on their own past experiences; they say to adolescents "enjoy these years while you can," "be glad you don't have to make decisions like we do," "you'll be grown soon enough and have to take on these responsibilities," "don't be in such a hurry to grow up," and "we don't want you to make the same mistakes we did." The "generation gap" describes the phenomenon in which the developmental tasks of these groups are in direct conflict with one another. Adolescents say, "let us grow and learn from our own decisions," and middle-aged adults say, "you can learn and benefit from the mistakes we made."

These generation differences are also expressed in the grieving process (see Table 2). The average adolescent has seen few deaths or major illnesses, whereas they are commonplace in the life of the middle-aged adult. Their differences in the perception of time is important. The adult in middle-age is able to appraise his feelings about his own mortality realistically. He has experienced grief and feels the pressure of time. His past is long, and the future is shorter. The passage of time seems rapid. The adolescent gives little attention to his own mortality; the past is short and the future is long. The trauma of grief is probably more unexpected for the adolescent than for the middle-aged adult. Life experience has little to do with grief time, but the grief processes at the two stages in life are in great contrast, much as are their developmental tasks.

The developmental stage of the health practitioner is significant in treating a grieving patient. In Figure 1, we diagram a hypothetical relationship between the grief experience of a health professional and an episode of grief in a patient. The middle line on the

TABLE 1

Developmental Tasks of Adolescence and Middle Adulthood*

Adolescence	Middle Adulthood
1. Achieving emotional indepedence of parents and other adults	1. Assisting teenage children to become responsible and happy adults
2. Accepting one's physique and using the body effectively	2. Accepting/adjusting to the physiological changes of middle age
3. Preparing for an economic career	3. Reaching/maintaining satisfactory performance in one's career
4. Desiring/achieving socially responsible behavior	4. Achieving adult civic and social responsibility
5. Achieving mature age-mate relationships with both sexes	5. Developing adult leisuretime activities
6. Achieving a masculine/ feminine role	6. Adjusting to aging parents
7. Preparing for marriage and family life	7. Relating oneself to one's mate as a person
8. Acquiring values/ethics as a guide to behavior; developing an ideology	

*See Havighurst

TABLE 2

Comparison of the Adolescent and Middle Adulthood Grieving Process*

Adolescence	Middle Adulthood
1. Grief due to death or illness is not common.	1. Grief due to death or illness is more common.
2. Grief is a distant and abstract event.	2. Grief is a realistic event.
3. Grief due to death or illness comes before its time; is untimely and unfair.	3. Grief due to death or illness comes as a natural cause of time; is part of the aging process.
4. Grief is tied with ideas of fate or circumstances of violence.	4. Grief is tied to realistic causes of real or symbolic loss.
5. Anger is at lost opportunities and ambitions.	5. Anger is at disruption of relationships and responsibilities towards others.
6. Here-and-now orientation to time results in an uncertainty about what to do with time that remains.	6. Past and future orientation to time results in a sense of time is running out.
7. Grief is something that happens to "others."	7. Grief is something that happens to "me."

*Adapted from Ambron, SR and Brodzindky, D: *Lifespan Human Development*. Holt, Rinehart and Winston: New York, 1979, pages 605-608.

Figure 1

Relationship Between the Hypothetical, Cumulative Grief Experience of a Health Professional and a Patient

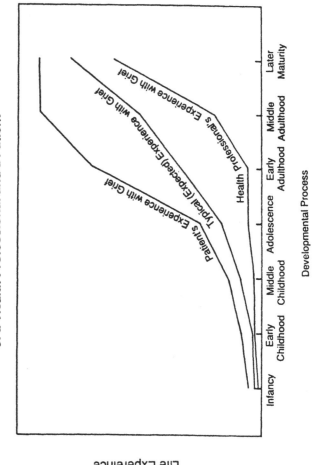

graph shows how a person with "average" life experience begins to acquire experience with grief in progressing through the developmental continuum. An individual's experience with grief is expected to increase with age, but the variability in experience as he or she progresses through the developmental continuum may be reflected in different perspectives of the health professional or the patient. The health practitioner must be aware of these differences to ensure that the evaluation and treatment process proceeds as effectively as possible.

A TEACHING MODEL

The course (or unit), depicted in Figure 2, is intended for a multidisciplinary group of allied health students, but it could also be useful to medical and nursing students. The student is introduced to concepts of human development described by such theorists as Havighurst (1979), Erikson (1963) and Piaget (1952). These theoretical concepts are integrated into a discussion of the specific developmental tasks for each life stage. The tasks of each stage are then evaluated in terms of the potential impact of trauma or disability, both generally and specifically.

The students learn about the grieving process: the definition of grieving, types of grieving, normal (versus "abnormal") grieving, behavioral responses, and adaptational patterns. The ideas of Kübler-Ross (1969), Worden (1982) and others are presented in terms of the concepts of developmental stages and tasks.

With a fundamental background of concepts of human development and the grief process, the students begin to apply this information to simulated patient situations, with themselves as the health care providers. The students are guided in the theoretical identification and analysis of patient needs, in terms of the individual's developmental stage and tasks. They must recognize the physical and mental adjustments or adaptations, real and symbolic, to loss of self or significant other(s). The students are then introduced to specific modes of assessing grieving patients. The degree of resolution of the tasks of mourning and the current place of the individual along the developmental continuum are identified and discussed in terms of the specific trauma, or disability, or the reason for impending

Figure 2

A Model for Teaching the Grief Process

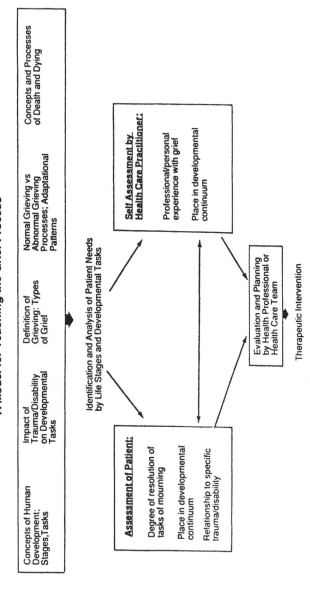

death. The potential role of a significant family member is also considered.

A key point in this educational process is that students recognize their own positions along the developmental continuum of professional and personal experiences—before any clinical interaction with the grieving patient. Therefore, as part of this course, they must practice self-assessment and identify their personal developmental stage, tasks, and coping behavior. They can then integrate patient data and data from their self-assessment to plan interactions in simulated patient situations. Actual therapeutic interventions are based on complete physical and mental evaluations and may involve a team of health practitioners. Other courses present the techniques for these evaluations and intervention strategies.

This course, however, provides a sound basis for understanding human development and the grieving process and their relationship to patient and self-assessment. It also provides a strong introduction to an important psychosocial dimension of clinical management. These concepts need to be developed further in more advanced didactic and clinically-based course work.

CONCLUSION

Several models for teaching about death and dying have been developed for medical education (Schoenberg et al. 1981). For the most part, these models are focused on specific courses on death and dying. We have taken the position that grief and grieving are part of life and not linked only to the event of death. Indeed, grief is a common human response to most physical and mental illnesses, especially chronic illnesses (Strauss, Corbin et al. 1984). Health professionals and patients have experiences with grief and illness as they progress through the life cycle. Our premise has been that health professionals can assist patients in the grief process and in the recovery from trauma if they have some understanding of their own attitudes and feelings about grief.

Learning about grief should be an integral part of the curriculum in all health professional schools. We have suggested that grief is a process itself and is part of human growth and development and, therefore, should be taught in human growth and development courses. Furthermore, teaching about grief should focus on its normal as well as its abnormal manifestations. Ideally, all types of health professionals should take such a course together, although it is not yet practical for this to occur. Although learning together does not ensure that health professionals will work together more effectively, it does increase the chance that they will have some understanding of one another's roles and of their common responsibility toward the patient.

A developmental approach to teaching students about the process of grieving acknowledges that it is a normal life experience and not limited to the event of death. Such an approach also implies that grieving individuals need understanding, support, and assistance from a variety of professionals if the resolution of grief and recovery or rehabilitation from illness is to occur.

REFERENCES

Bridle, M. (1977). "Death: A topic for occupational therapy curricula." *Canadian Journal of Occupational Therapy, 44*, 71-72.

Bruhn, J. G. (1981). "Death and dying in the life cycle." In B. Schoenberg et al. (Eds.). *The Education of the Medical Student in Thanatology*. New York: Arno Press.

Dickens, D. N. & Mullen, J. (1983). "Confronting death and dying: Training for clinical dieticians." *Journal of the American Dietetic Association, 83*, 690-692.

Dietrich, M. C. (1980). "A proposed curriculum on death and dying for the allied health student." *Journal of Allied Health, 9*, 25-32.

Erikson, E. H. (1963). *Childhood and Society*. Second Edition. New York: W. W. Norton and Co.

Gammage, S. L., McMahon, P. S. & Shanahan, P. M. (1976). "Learning to cope with death." *American Journal of Occupational Therapy, 30*, 294-299.

Goldstein, E. (1977). "Teaching social work perspective on the dying patient and his family." In E. Prichard, J. Collard, B. Arcuth, A. Kutscher, I. Seeland and H. Lefkloutz (Eds.). *Social Work With the Dying Patient and the Family*. New York: Columbia University Press.

Harris, A. P. (1980). "Content and method in a thanatology training program for paraprofessionals." *Death Education, 4*, 21-27.

Havighurst, R. J. (1979). *Developmental Tasks and Education*. Third Edition. New York: David McKay.

Kaluger, G. and Kaluger, M. F. (1984). *Human Development — The Span of Life*. Third Edition. Time Mirror/ Mosby Publishing.

Kübler-Ross, E. (1969). *On Death and Dying*. New York: Macmillan.

Lutticken, C. A., Shepard, K. F. & Davies, N. R. (1974). "Attitudes of physical therapists toward death and illness." *Physical Therapy*, *54*, 226-232.

Miller, R. (1977). "Teaching death and dying content in the social work curriculum." In E. Prichard, J. Collard, B. Arcuth, A. Kutscher, I. Seeland and H. Lefkloutz (Eds.). *Social Work With the Dying Patient and the Family*. New York: Columbia University Press.

Piaget, J. (1952). *The Origins of Intelligence in Children*. New York: International Universities Press.

Purtilo, R. B. (1972). "Don't mention it: The physical therapist in a death-denying society." *Physical Therapy*, *52*, 1031-1035.

Schoenberg, B., Carr, A. C., Kutscher, A. H., Mark, L. C., DeBellis, R., Peretz, D. and Gerber, I. (Eds.). (1981). *Education of the Medical Student in Thanatology*. New York: Arno Press.

Simon, I. T. (1971). "Emotional aspects of physical disability." *The American Journal of Occupational Therapy*, *25*, 408-410.

Sinacore, J. M. (1981). "Avoiding the humanistic aspect of death: An outcome from the implicit elements of health professions education." *Death Education*, *5*, 121-133.

Stewart, T. D. & Rossier, A. B. (1978). "Psychological considerations in the adjustment to spinal cord injury." *Rehabilitation Literature*, *39*, 75-80.

Strauss, A. L., Corbin, J. et al. (1984). *Chronic Illness and the Quality of Life*. Second Edition. St. Louis: Mosby.

Worden, J. W. (1982). *Grief Counseling and Grief Therapy*. New York: Springer Publishing Co.

Zelinsky, L. F. & Thorson, J. A. (1983). "Educational approaches to preparing social work students for practice related to death and dying." *Death Education*, *6*, 313-322.

Implementation of the Management of the Grieving Process in the Curriculum at Suffolk Community College

Mary A. Crosley
Sister Mary Ann Borello

The nursing program at Suffolk Community College in Brentwood, New York, is a two-year course leading to an associate degree in applied science. The faculty has selected Maslow's Hierarchy of Needs (Kozier and Erb 1983) as the conceptual framework, and nursing process and nursing diagnoses as two of the major threads. It is within this framework that students begin to understand the dying patient and the grieving process. From that point, appropriate interventions can be developed.

The clinical rotations include acute care, community-oriented hospitals with a high percentage of elderly patients. An oncology unit is also included in the rotations. This combination means that even first-semester students may have direct practice with patients and families experiencing the grieving process.

The beginning student is introduced to the stages of bereavement during the first semester. The objectives are to have the students know those stages, the normal emotional response to loss, and the fears that the dying patient experiences.

The first stage of bereavement is characterized by denial. Family and close friends are still very emotionally involved with the dying person and are not ready "to let the person go." The middle stage of disorganization is a time of disequilibrium within the family system. Emotional energy attached to the dying person is being released. The family's grief is in the process of being resolved but it is not resolved sufficiently to invest emotional energy elsewhere. It is a very unsettling time and it is not unusual to question one's own

93

sanity at this time. The stage of reorganization is characterized by being able to reinvest emotional energy and being able to experience emotional gratification from a new situation.

Fears the dying person may experience include fear of the unknown, of loneliness, of sorrow, of loss of body, of loss of self-control, of suffering and pain, of identity, and of regression. The students are encouraged to help patients and families verbalize their fears. They are then guided in developing nursing care plans that address the individual's specific fears.

This aspect of the curriculum is taught in didactic form with student discussion included to the extent that time permits. During the second semester, small group discussions of 10-11 students further explore the death and dying process. A two-hour college lab is devoted to this topic.

The students are first introduced to the nursing process and nursing diagnosis at the end of the first semester. These are expanded in the clinical area and during the college lab on the Grieving Process. Here they are helped to identify the cues of coping patterns that are ineffective and to plan intervention. The students are guided in learning the normal emotional response to loss, the effects on the grieving person of the social environment, and the identification of adaptive and maladaptive coping mechanisms.

The Nursing Diagnosis identified by the North American Nursing Diagnosis Association (NANDA) (Carpenito 1983) is utilized. The student is taught to identify subjective and objective assessment data that are related to the anticipated loss, to establish outcome criteria that will be expected following nursing intervention, and to implement specific interventions. This is accomplished through the framework of nursing diagnosis. A valuable resource in this area is *Nursing Diagnosis Application to Clinical Practice* by Lynda Carpenito (1983). Some nursing diagnoses that are applicable to the dying patient and the family members are:

- Coping, ineffective individual (and/or family);
- Family processes alteration in relation to an ill family member;
- Grieving related to actual or perceived loss;
- Grieving related to anticipated loss.

Also, in the second semester, the students learn the mental health component of the curriculum. Communication skills, interviewing, and counseling techniques are discussed. They identify early clues of suicide and explore suicide prevention.

During the third semester, the students study Maternal-Child Nursing from the individual and family points of view. One aspect of the clinical focus and clinical worksheets is the specific concentration on SIDS (Sudden Infant Death Syndrome). The community agencies available as resources for patients and families are examined.

In the maternal nursing theory component, students identify the woman's and family's reactions to miscarriage and the elective termination of pregnancy. Students are encouraged to explore their own feelings on these emotionally charged issues. The nurse's role in counseling the individual and the family is discussed.

The fourth semester provides the student with the clinical opportunity to integrate the theory regarding the grieving process in the clinical area. One clinical rotation is on a medical oncology unit. Here the students experience the value of support groups. The hospital has pastoral visitors, a thanatology team, and supportive clinical nurses who have studied oncology. The thanatology team not only helps the hospitalized patient but the patient's family as well. The team also makes follow-up calls and home visits after the individual's death. The students benefit from the excellent clinical role models.

The fourth semester is the advanced medical-surgical experience, including a brief introduction into critical care areas. The high acuity of patient illness demands that the students can identify appropriate and inappropriate responses in anticipatory grieving and can assist the patient and family to identify helpful interventions. Once this step is accomplished, the student can use supporting positive coping mechanisms.

During the fourth semester, the students have the option of rotating through the Emergency Department. Here they have the opportunity to help patients and/or family members faced with sudden, traumatic events, such as sudden heart attacks and severe auto accidents. When the medical problem is the result of attempted suicide or homicide, the emotional responses are heightened. Here the students are introduced to legal reporting and recording policies.

In addition to the required work described above, the student also has the option of selecting a 3-credit social science elective on Death and Dying. This course is taught by Mary Ann Borello, Professor of Sociology. This course examines the cultural, religious, and social milieus in which support groups form during the grieving process. The development of this course was jointly supported by nursing and social science faculty. It is open to all college students.

In the Death and Dying course, students explore the American response to death. They examined some behaviors of Americans that indicate denial of death. They develop a cross-cultural perspective by comparing the Puerto Rican culture with the American culture.

The teaching format encourages active participation and sharing of individual feelings, reactions, and experiences. Students are introduced to the topic by active exercises. The first day's homework is to share the fact that they are taking a death and dying course with family and friends. At the next class meeting, all students report the responses that they encountered.

Teaching methods focus on the theories of research in sociology and anthropology. This is balanced with active exercises that provide the focus for student discussion and participation. Some of the exercises follow.

1. *Amount of exposure.* Members of the group are asked to share their individual direct experiences with a dying person. The number of funerals attended as well as the age group of the individual and the deceased are discussed. Number and timing of visits to the cemetery and one's feelings about visiting grave sites are explored.

2. *Reporting of death.* The class is asked to review the daily newspaper to note the coverage of death. How and what types of death get reported on the front page or in the narrative section? How do these stories differ from the coverage on the obituary page?

3. *Children's fairy tales.* The student selects a well-known children's fairy tale and analyzes how the tale describes and por-

trays death. One fairy tale frequently chosen is "Sleeping Beauty."

4. *Preparing for dying*. The practical aspects of life insurance and preparing a will as well as the motivating and restraining forces that surround these activities are discussed.

5. *Role play*. The student is asked to assume the role of a physician who is telling an individual that he or she is dying. Following this, the student assumes the role of the dying person. Students are asked to focus on where they want to die, who would be with them during the dying process, what staff and health professionals would be available, and what decorations and symbols would be around them. Whom would they want in their support systems?

6. *Cancer patient*. Students imagine they are terminally ill cancer patients. They share what people say to them and how they communicate. What topics are "safe" to discuss? The type of gifts and "get well" cards people give are discussed. How do family and friends touch the dying person? Is it distant or close and intimate? The frequency and length of visits are discussed.

A student who takes this course is a different individual upon completing the course. He or she is more sensitized to the needs of the dying person.

Nursing students at Suffolk Community College have the opportunity to examine the grieving process during the entire four semesters. They begin by identifying the assessment parameters and progress to complex intervention and evaluation plans. The program provides students with support and time during their training to become more sophisticated in their personal and professional management of the grieving process.

REFERENCES

Carpenito, L. (1983). *Nursing Diagnosis Application to Clinical Practice*. Philadelphia: J. P. Lippincott.

Kozier, B. and Erb, G. (1983). *Fundamentals of Nursing Concepts and Procedures*. California: Addison Wesley.

Clinical Imperatives versus Ethical Commitments in Euthanasia: The Perspectives of Nurses

Mostafa H. Nagi

Once medically defined as such, terminal illness describes a change in the status of illness from that of expected recovery to that of impending death. The literature abounds with reports of the role conflict medical professionals are increasingly confronting in treating terminally ill patients. Technological advances, material costs, the moral and religious feelings of the patient, family pressure, and fear of legal risks all create severe conflict for physicians (Brown et al. 1970; Flew 1970; Levine and Scotch 1970). Medical education, with its lack of preparation for caring for the dying patient and its firm dedication to the saving of life at any cost, is a major source of internal conflict (Handin 1973; Weisman 1972). Currently, it appears that the medical imperative of sustaining all life, regardless of costs, may be the more encompassing force acting on the physician (Ramsey 1970, 1972).

Research evidence, however, strongly indicates that whether physicians are in favor of forms of euthanasia or not they must

99

make life-sustaining decisions. These decisions are, therefore, usually made with a large degree of variance (Crane 1973; G. Fletcher 1970; J. Fletcher 1970). Until recently, the medical profession has not actively sought solutions to this dilemma, but euthanasia has become a subject of considerable concern in recent years and there is every indication of a growing controversy surrounding it (Kluge 1981; Horan and Mall 1977; and Grisez and Boyle 1979).

Sol Levine and Norman Scotch (1970) conclude that, "the power of the new technology to maintain life considerably beyond the patient's capacity to function socially emphasizes the need to reexamine and reassess the application of religious and legal norms which govern the lifesaving role of the physician" (p. 221).

Similar to the doctor, the nurse is educated in the current philosophy of the Hippocratic Oath, which singularly focuses on the patient's improvement in health (Maguire 1974; Friedson 1971; Freeman et al. 1970). Eliot Friedson notes, "indeed, in the Hippocratic corpus it was suggested that the physician's apprentice be left behind at the bedside to carry out the doctor's orders in a more reliable way than could be expected of the patient or his family" (p. 58). Therefore, the nurse is expected to carry out the doctor's orders to heal, but unlike the doctor, she constantly observes the suffering patients endure before she can ease pain and anguish. Despite close contact with the dying patient, and although she may feel bereavement, discouragement, and depression, her role is not usually amenable to the expression of grief (Popoff 1975; Glaser 1965).

The strains on the nurse's role are further accentuated by the fact that, while she is given numerous responsibilities, her authority in many respects is limited. If one adds to that her close association with the terminal patient and family, as well as her dual role as their source of communication with the physician and vice versa, the nurse's dilemma becomes clear. Glaser and Strauss (1968) observe that nurses are often the ones who actually sustain life or permit death, either on orders from the doctor or because of their own inclinations.

Whether nurses are in favor of forms of euthanasia or not, their work requires them to perform life-sustaining acts. Turning off the respirator is perhaps the most dramatic act of euthanasia by omission. Nursing acts of euthanasia by omission are not always dependent on physician's orders. Nursing acts of omission might include *not* turning a comatose, terminal patient every two hours, *not* withholding morphine when respiratory failure is suspected, *not* providing sensory stimulation, *not* forcing oral intake, *not* encouraging ambulation, and *not* recording intake and output. Not performing these acts could be interpreted as a form of passive euthanasia. In brief, a nurse could question whether or not she is prolonging the inevitable for a terminal patient when she performs what is considered acceptable nursing care.

It is generally recognized that nurses' striving toward professional status is in many respects linked to the conflict between their role and that of the physician (Pellegrino 1964; Bates 1972; Meyer and Hoffman 1964).

Contemporary trends toward professionalization in nursing (Schulman 1972; Hogstel 1977; Reeder and Haus 1979) led us to hypothesize that nurses view themselves increasingly as professionals who are entitled to make their own assessments of medical practice and who reserve the right to evaluate critically the practices of physicians.

The nurses' separate and distinct skills and experience in caring, comforting, counseling, and helping patients and their families cope with their health problems (Smoyak 1974) stand in contrast with the physician's experience in diagnosing and curing of disease. When the two professionals deal with the terminally ill patient, the conflict between their roles becomes more apparent.

Referring specifically to euthanasia, this study provides a test for the following: (1) the nurses' perspective on the degree of congruency between their professional roles and the role of physicians in dealing with terminally ill patients, and (2) the nurses' readiness to translate their expressed attitudes into nursing practices.

In and outside the medical professions, euthanasia is clearly recognized to be a highly controversial issue (Carlton 1980; Carney 1979; Downing 1970; Meyers 1970; and Nagi 1977, 1980, and 1982). Clinically, a major concern in such controversy centers around the use of "life-sustaining" instruments, the use of "pain-killing drugs," and the possibility of miracle cures.

Probing the nurses' opinions on these matters, we believed, could refine attitudinal expressions among the respondents and thus shed greater light on the test of the hypothesis. Accordingly, nurses in the sample were first asked to respond to a number of questions related to the use of life-sustaining instruments. Second, nurses were asked to express their views on the use of pain-killing drugs to alleviate the suffering of some terminally ill patients. Respondents were also asked their opinions concerning the need to prolong the life of the dying patient because of the possibility of a miracle cure.

SAMPLE AND BACKGROUND DATA

The data reported here were drawn from a much larger probability sample of nurses and clergy in the state of Ohio. Four hundred thirty-nine nurses were selected from the directory obtained from the Ohio Nursing Board Association. The return rate for the mailed questionnaire was 184 (43 percent) after two follow-ups of the original questionnaire at approximately two-week intervals.[1] The questionnaire sent to the nurses consisted of five parts. Preceding each section, significant terms were defined and instructions were specified to help ensure uniformity of response. Part I elicited approval or disapproval of a number of statements related to the experience of the terminal patient, especially the desire for easy and dignified death. Part II consisted of a set of items which specified certain conditions under which passive and active voluntary euthanasia could be considered morally permissible. Part III included items related to legalization of euthanasia and the need to establish legal guidelines.

The fourth part of the questionnaire focused on the professional role of the nurse and the duties and the rights that go with the role, especially as these are related to the physician's role in matters concerned with the dying patient. The last part of the questionnaire included items concerning background variables such as age, marital status, religion, and the size of the community of origin. A sec-

---

1. The reader should be aware that the statistical results in this pilot study may have some margins of error resulting from the relatively low response rates of the nurses to the mailed questionnaire which pertained to these highly sensitive and controversial issues.

ond group of variables included the degree of education, medical specialization and practices, occupational duties, etc.

A description of the socioeconomic characteristics of the 189 respondents included: Age: 24% were classified as young (23 to 35 years), 41% were middle aged (36 to 49 years), and 35% were categorized as old (50 to 85 years); Size of Home Community: 30% was rural (less than 2,000), 26% was town (2,000-25,000), and 44% was urban (more than 25,000); Religion: 39% were Catholic, 61% were Protestants); Education: 38% had no four-year degree (diploma or associate degree), 31% had a Bachelor's degree in nursing, 15% had a Bachelor's degree in Liberal Arts, and 16% had Masters degrees; Marital Status: 17% were single, 71% were married, 12% were widowed or divorced; Parent's Class Position: 61% were middle class and 39% were working class; and Father's Occupation: 31% were professional-managerial, 14% were white collar (salesworkers and clerks), 35% were blue collar (skilled and unskilled workers) and 20% were farmers.

The occupational backgrounds of the respondents were as follows: Medical specialty: 32% were geriatric and 68% nongeriatric; Type of Position: 18% were administrators or consultants, 16% were supervisors, 21% were instructors, 15% were head nurses, and 30% were general duty nurses; and Field of Nursing Practice: 37% were in hospital, 24% were in nursing home, 18% were in school of nursing, and 21% of the nurses were in nonhospital related employment (e.g., school nurse, industrial nurse, public health nurse).

DATA ANALYSIS

Euthanasia Forms and Acceptable Conditions

A preliminary issue is the question of distinguishing between different forms of euthanasia. Euthanasia can occur because of an act of commission or an act of omission—a refusal to act. Euthanasia by omission at the request of a patient of sound mind is not a crucial issue; the patient now has the right to decline treatment or any further treatment. The term voluntary euthanasia refers more properly to acts of commission requested by a legally responsible adult. Two types of voluntary euthanasia can be differentiated: active voluntary euthanasia and passive voluntary euthanasia. Passive voluntary euthanasia involves an act which permits natural death (e.g., the discontinuance of life-supporting treatment), while active voluntary euthanasia involves an act which directly induces death (e.g., the prescription of a lethal dose of some substance). Subsequent discussion maintains this distinction and presupposes that terminal illness (illness leading to death despite treatment within six months) can be determined with reasonable certainty.

The importance of the ethical distinction between passive and active voluntary euthanasia is especially manifest in the attitudes of the nurses. In this regard, the respondents were asked to indicate whether or not they believed passive voluntary euthanasia (the discontinuance of life-supporting treatment) should be granted an incurably ill terminal patient in each of eight different circumstances. The nurses were requested to view these items through the perspective of the terminal patient. Five of the eight conditions were also appropriate for voluntary active euthanasia. Table 1 allows easy comparison of responses.

The Guttman scale technique was used to determine the order of appearance of the items. The eight items scaled with a highly acceptable coefficient of reproducibility of .88. All items scaled and, therefore, no deletions were necessary to attain the desired ordering of statements. Thus, we made the assumption that the statements are aligned along some latent structural dimension. This dimension, on a manifest level, reveals varying degrees of tolerance toward passive voluntary euthanasia. The specified conditions are assumed to form an accumulative dimension. One could, therefore, expect that, for example, if an individual does not approve of passive euthanasia because of the first condition ("The patient wants to go home and die in peace with his family"), he would not approve of passive euthanasia in any of the other seven conditions. Stated another way, if the lowest condition approved by a nurse is number five, it can be expected that she approves of passive euthanasia in conditions one through four but not conditions six through eight.

The findings reveal that the assumption that nurses are generally opposed to passive euthanasia because of their dedication to healing is not substantiated. In fact, the findings suggest that they strongly

TABLE 1. Acceptance of Attitutes Toward Passive and Active Euthanasia in Specified Circumstances

Condition	Passive Euthanasia				Active Euthanasia			
	A	UD	UA	N	A	UD	UA	N
1. The patient wants to die in peace at home	75*	6	19	180	(-)	(-)	(-)	(-)
2. The patient feels the pain and psychological strain are intolerable	72	10	18	179	7	12	71	177
3. The patient has special reasons of conscience	57	11	32	179	(-)	(-)	(-)	(-)
4. The patient feels undignified or demeaned by his medical condition	54	20	26	180	13	17	70	180
5. The patient doesn't want to live any longer	52	17	31	179	15	17	68	179
6. The patient feels it prolongs psychological stress on his family	46	21	33	178	0	16	77	180
7. The patient feels the cost of his treatment is a severe financial hardship for his family	44	25	31	180	7	17	76	179
8. The patient has personal reasons --family, spiritual, etc.--for retaining consciousness and mental acuity	42	11	46	178	(-)	(-)	(-)	(-)

*The numbers listed in response categories are percentages.

A = acceptable
UD = undecided
UA = unacceptable

tolerate euthanasia under specific conditions. The distinction they made between active and passive euthanasia is quite clear. They find passive euthanasia to be quite acceptable, under most conditions, but active euthanasia to be much less acceptable.

Note that 75% of the nurses find passive euthanasia acceptable if the "patient wants to die in peace at home with his family." The emphasis on death with dignity is manifest. The condition that rates second, "if pain and psychological strain are intolerable" is given much the same acceptance. Human dignity, physical and emotional pain are rated highly by the nurses as justifications for passive euthanasia. Therefore, they appear to be against the prolongation of physical life under all conditions.

The nurses in the sample appear not to be as concerned about family members as about the patient. Thus "psychological stress on the family" is ranked *seventh*.

It may be concluded that nurses tend to be patient-oriented in their ordering of the justifications for passive euthanasia. They place more emphasis on clinical matters including physical and emotional comfort of the patient and tend to deemphasize reasons that are peripheral to the patient's well-being. Thus, financial and pyschological costs to the family are not given priority nor are reasons viewed as imposed on the patient by the family or church. However, the patient's own desires for comfort are given precedence. Thus, the following conditions, ranked third, fourth, and fifth, respectively, take precedence over external pressures: "The patient has special reasons for conscience," "the patient feels undignified or demeaned by his condition," and "the patient doesn't want to live any longer." Yet, they rank below the personal pain and strain of the patient.

Protestant and Catholic nurses tend to have similar attitudes toward passive euthanasia. The nurses of the two faiths almost always find the conditions for passive euthanasia more acceptable than unacceptable (Table 2). There is only one exception. Catholic nurses find statement eight, the patient has personal reasons for retaining consciousness and mental acuity, more unacceptable (52 percent) than acceptable (38 percent).

However, when comparing Catholic responses with Protestant, it should be noted that the percentage of Protestant "acceptable" responses always exceeded the percentage of Catholic "acceptable" responses for each condition and the percentage of "unacceptable" Catholic responses always exceeded the percentage of Protestant "unacceptable" responses for each condition. Furthermore, this Protestant-Catholic differential can be judged statistically significant, by using either the chi square or the gamma correlation in six of the eight items.

The differential responses between the two religions are even more pronounced when referring to active euthanasia. Table 2 illustrates that of the five conditions presented to the nurses for active euthanasia, all manifested highly significant chi squares and gamma correlations. A review of the responses illustrated, once again, that Protestants are significantly more accepting of active euthanasia in a comparison of each acceptable or unacceptable category within each condition. Although Protestants are much more accepting of active euthanasia, they are generally opposed to the practice.

One can conceivably argue that nurses who are in medical specialties closely involved with the care of the terminally ill may be more opposed to euthanasia because of the sympathies they develop toward the patient. However, another line of argument may start with the idea that those close to the suffering, terminal patients may want to see their suffering painlessly ended. Table 3 compares geriatric with nongeriatric nurses on conditions acceptable for passive and active euthanasia.[2]

The table illustrates some of the data bearing on this controversy. Geriatric nurses are significantly more opposed to passive euthanasia than nongeriatric nurses. Only the first statement, "Patient wants to die in peace at home with his family," is found more acceptable by the geriatric nurses. This statement places emphasis on the happiness of the final days of the patient and may indicate

---

2. The dichotomy between geriatric and nongeriatric specializations may be somewhat superficial. However, we assumed that geriatric nurses would be more likely to be faced with decisions regarding passive and active euthanasia than nongeriatric nurses. We are aware, however, that by making this assumption we may have overlooked a great deal of data regarding nurses working in neonatal intensive care, adult intensive care, oncological and terminal care settings where nurses question their attitudes toward euthanasia regardless of the age of the patient population.

TABLE 2. Conditions Acceptable for Passive and Active Euthanasia by Religion

Passive Euthanasia

	Catholics			
	A	UD	UA	N
1. Die with family	63	8	29	51
2. Intolerable pain and psychologial strain	58	13	29	52
3. Special reasons for conscience	43	16	41	51
4. Undignified or demeaned by medical condition	46	21	33	52
5. Patient doesn't want to live any longer	44	19	37	52
6. Prolongs psychological stress on family	44	21	35	52
7. Cost of treatment is severe financial hardship	46	21	33	52
8. Personal reasons for retaining consciousness and mental acuity	38	10	52	52

A = acceptable
UD = undecided
UA = unacceptable

Degrees of freedom = 2

+ Values in X^2 colums are expressed as significance levels.
The numbers listed in response categories are percentages.

that geriatric nurses feel an institution is not a good place for the elderly to spend their final days. The question must be asked, to what extent do geriatric nurses experience the suffering of terminal patients? In addition, we must ask if geriatric nurses disapprove of passive euthanasia to a greater extent than nongeriatric nurses because they fear that euthanasia may spread and abuses may especially affect the elderly.

The geriatric/nongeriatric attitudinal differential is present, but to a lesser extent, when considering active euthanasia. Although geri-

Passive Euthanasia				X^2+	gamma	Active Euthanasia								X^2	gamma
Protestants						Catholics				Protestants					
A	UD	UA	N			A	UD	UA	N	A	UD	UA	N		
82	5	13	119	019	.45	(-)	(-)	(-)	(-)	(-)	(-)	(-)	(-)	(-)	(-)
78	8	14	118	023	.42	4	6	90	51	20	15	65	117	.003	.65
61	9	30	119	084	.29	(-)	(-)	(-)	(-)	(-)	(-)	(-)	(-)	(-)	(-)
58	18	24	119	330	.21	8	8	83	52	14	20	66	119	.038	.44
56	16	28	117	331	.21	8	8	84	51	18	19	63	119	.022	.48
48	20	32	117	901	.06	2	6	92	52	9	21	70	119	.006	.66
46	25	29	119	797	.04	4	6	90	52	9	21	70	118	.013	.58
46	13	41	116	437	.17	(-)	(-)	(-)	(-)	(-)	(-)	(-)	(-)	(-)	(-)

atric nurses are more opposed to active euthanasia than nongeriatric nurses, the two nursing categories show a relatively strong feeling in opposition to active euthanasia.

The Nurse's Perspective on Her Role
in Relationship to the Physician's Role

As shown in Table 4, 64 percent of the respondents agree that "Nurses are just as qualified as physicians to make decisions concerning medical ethics;" only 22 percent disagree. Eighty-one percent of the nurses disagree (50 percent strongly) that ". . . the duties of the nurse are only and primarily to carry out the doctor's orders." Nurses tend to view themselves as professionals in their own right, capable of disagreeing with the actions of the physician.

Referring specifically to euthanasia, the majority of nurses indicate they should have the right to request an inquiry by a medical

TABLE 3. Conditions Acceptable for Passive and Active Euthanasia by Medical Specialization

	Passive Euthanasia Geriatric Non-geriatric			
	A	UD	UA	N
1. Die with family	79	9	12	58
2. Intolerable pain and psychologial strain	69	12	19	59
3. Special reasons for conscience	48	17	35	58
4. Undignified or demeaned by medical condition	44	17	39	59
5. Patient doesn't want to live any longer	45	15	40	58
6. Prolongs psychological stress on family	39	22	39	59
7. Cost of treatment is severe financial hardship	32	29	39	59
8. Personal reasons for retaining consciousness and mental acuity	38	21	41	58

A = acceptable
UD = undecided
UA = unacceptable

Degrees of freedom = 2

+ Values in X^2 colums are expressed as significance levels.
The numbers listed in response categories are percentages.

board if they feel a patient qualifies for voluntary euthanasia but the attending physician does not (item 3). Statements four and five, however, both ask the nurse if she should "carry out the physician's order," but statement four refers to the order to "hasten death" and item five to the command to "discontinue life-sustaining measures." In addition, this statement on passive euthanasia includes a signed patient or next of kin waiver. The nurses are much less op-

Passive Euthanasia Geriatric Non-geriatric				x^{2+}	gamma	Active Euthanasia Geriatric Non-geriatric								x^2	gamma
A	UD	UA	N			A	UD	UA	N	A	UD	UA	N		
74	7	19	62	.523	.16	(-)	(-)	(-)	(-)	(-)	(-)	(-)	(-)	(-)	(-)
82	5	13	61	.231	.30	(-)	(-)	(-)	(-)	(-)	(-)	(-)	(-)	(-)	(-)
66	5	29	62	.045	.25	(-)	(-)	(-)	(-)	(-)	(-)	(-)	(-)	(-)	(-)
68	19	13	62	.004	.47	10	14	76	59	15	14	71	62	.742	.14
62	18	20	61	.054	.35	12	10	78	59	19	15	66	62	.345	.27
57	24	19	62	.050	.35	5	14	81	59	10	18	72	62	.473	.24
60	22	18	62	.006	.46	5	14	81	58	8	18	74	62	.653	.19
55	3	42	62	.008	.16	(-)	(-)	(-)	(-)	(-)	(-)	(-)	(-)	(-)	(-)

posed (73 percent agreed compared to 14 percent opposed) to "discontinuing life-sustaining measures" with a "signed waiver by the next of kin" (statement 5) than they are of "hastening death" (item 4) by the physician's order" (42 percent in favor in comparison to 36 percent opposed). Passive euthanasia, when accompanied by a signed waiver, seems to be more acceptable to nurses.

The independence expressed by the nurses in this sample in such matters as medical ethics is further substantiated by the overwhelming agreement among nurses (statement 6) that even if legal guidelines are established it is the prerogative of the individual nurse to refuse to carry out the legal orders with which she disagrees (87 percent take this position).

Ordinarily, one might not expect religion to be a differentiating factor in the nurse's perspective of her role in relationship to the

TABLE 4. Nurse's Role in Relationship to the Physician's Role

		Total Response					
		SA	A	U	D	SD	N
1.	Nurses are as qualified as physicians to make ethics decisions	20	*44	14	20	2	177
2.	The duties of the nurse are only to carry out the doctor's orders	4	10	5	31	50	182
3.	The nurse should be able to request an inquiry by a medical board for patient's voluntary euthanasia	11	43	16	21	9	180
4.	With legal approval the nurse should carry out doctor's orders to hasten death	6	36	22	23	13	178
5.	Nurses should follow physician's order to discontinue life support if there is signed waiver from patient	13	60	13	8	6	179
6.	Nurses should have the right to refuse to carry out order for euthanasia even if it is legal	46	41	6	7	0	179

* The numbers listed in response categories are percentages.

SA = strongly agree
 A = agree
 U = undecided
 D = disagree
SD = strongly disagree

physician's role. Yet, most items in Table 5 shows some measure of significant differentation by religious affiliation.

Catholic nurses seem to be more ready to argue that the nurse has the right to refuse to carry out the doctor's orders. It may be that Catholic nurses have become more sensitized to their rights since, especially with respect to abortion, they have been confronted, more than Protestant nurses, with the likelihood of having to carry out physicians' orders which may be contrary to their convictions. This rationale may also explain why Catholic nurses may have slightly stronger feelings about being just as qualified as physicians to make decisions in medical ethics (Table 5, statement one). However, the Protestant nurses agree, to a significantly greater extent than Catholics, that a nurse has the right to request an inquiry by a medical board if she believes a patient qualifies for voluntary euthanasia but the attending physician does not.

Perhaps Catholic nurses are more sensitized to issues relating to potential violations of their own moral code whereas the Protestant nurses may focus more attention on the potential abuses of euthanasia by the physician. These conclusions are not meant to ignore that, generally, both Protestant and Catholic nurses have similar opinions of their professional role vis-à-vis the physician, but their perceptions of the issues do appear to be shaped significantly by their religious backgrounds.

Table 5 shows that geriatric nurses tend to be more opposed to most of the statements which suggest that the nurse should have the authority to act independently of the physician's orders. Only two statements (4 and 5) did not produce appreciable differentiation, although they tended to show percentages in the expected direction. The two nursing categories responded similarly to the items which suggested that nurses should carry out the physician's order for passive euthanasia. Thus, statements denoting more sensitive issues surrounding the nurse's prerogative to act independently of the physician invited greater differences in opinion between the two groups of nurses.

Perspectives on Clinical Practices: The Maintenance of Life-Sustaining Instruments, the Use of Pain-Killing Drugs and the Possibility of Miracle Cure

The growth of medical technology has led to a proliferation of techniques for life-sustaining instruments. The nurse has assumed the distinct role of continuously supervising the functioning of these

TABLE 5. Nurse's Role in Relationship to the Physician's Role

	Catholic						Protestant					
	SA	A	U	D	SD	N	SA	A	U	D	SD	N
1. Nurses are as qualified as physicians to make ethics decisions	25	45	18	12	0	51	20	43	12	22	3	117
2. The duties of the nurse are only to carry on the doctor's orders	8	2	4	36	50	52	2	13	4	31	50	120
3. The nurse should be able to request an inquiry by a medical board for patient's voluntary euthanasia	18	23	18	25	16	51	9	51	15	19	6	119
4. With legal approval the nurse should carry out doctor's orders to hasten death	2	14	29	31	24	51	8	46	19	19	8	117
5. Nurses should follow physician's order to discontinue life support if there is signed waiver from patient	8	57	13	12	10	51	16	61	13	7	3	118
6. Nurses should have the right to refuse to carry out order for euthanasia even if it is legal	69	27	2	0	2	51	37	45	8	10	0	118

Degrees of freedom = 4

+ Values in X^2 columns are expressed as significance levels.
The numbers listed in response categories are percentages.

instruments, whether on her own initiative or when she is carrying out the doctor's orders. Therefore, the nurse's views on the maintenance of these instruments are of prime importance in consideration of both her first-hand knowledge of them and her essential role in their operation.

As Table 6 indicates, nurses tend to disagree that renal hemodialysis (a medical process that fulfills the kidney's functions by the periodic removal of wastes from the blood) that would prolong life should always be continued *if the patient has adequate funds*. The patient's ability to incur cost is perhaps the qualification that may have led to the strongly unfavorable response to this item. The sec-

x^2+	Gamma	Geriatric						Non-geriatric						x^2+	Gamma
		SA	A	U	D	SD	N	SA	A	U	D	SD	N		
.264	.19	14	36	20	25	5	59	25	48	10	17	0	60	.052	.37
.063	.03	8	19	10	29	34	59	0	3	0	40	57	62	.000	.53
.009	.20	3	46	14	24	13	59	20	40	25	12	3	60	.004	.36
.000	.53	5	37	20	24	14	59	3	40	24	23	10	60	.949	.04
.220	.30	10	63	14	8	5	59	12	60	11	12	5	60	.975	.01
.000	.55	41	37	8·	14	0	59	50	42	5	1	2	60	.099	.25

ond statement reveals, however, that nurses are willing to give significant consideration to the desires of the family regardless of cost.

Nurses reject the argument for the continuation of life-supporting efforts if the patient has adequate funds, yet they are willing to maintain life, regardless of cost, if the family so requests. It appears that nurses tend to place greater importance on personal and family factors than on factors of cost in the maintenance of life-supporting instruments.

Statements three and four address the issue of the request of a patient or responsible relative for passive euthanasia. This set of items produces fewer undecided responses than the statements pertaining to the more complex factor of cost. Eighty-eight percent agree that "terminal patients should be free to request and receive passive euthanasia without fear of legal sanction." Nurses also tend to agree (58 percent) with the last statement, which asserts that a

TABLE 6. Perspective on Clinical Issues Related to the Terminal Patient

Statement	Response*					
	SA	A	U	D	SD	N
A. Maintenance of Life-Sustaining Instruments						
1. Knowing that renal hemodialysis would prolong life, it should always be continued as treatment for those patients with adequate funds	9	24	20	34	13	177
2. Life sustaining treatment to the suffering terminal patient should be maintained if the family demands treatment be continued regardless of cost	5	45	27	20	3	181
3. Terminal patients should be free to request and receive passive euthanasia without fear of legal sanction	34	54	6	4	2	181
4. A signed waiver of the patient or responsible relative should be necessary for the passive euthanasia of a patient expected to die in a few days	8	50	13	23	6	176

B. The use of Pain-Killing Drugs

	SA	A	U	D	SD	
1. It is right for a physician to order pain and consciousness removing drugs for a terminal patient even though the drug may shorten life	23	60	10	6	2	181
2. Patients should have the right to request and receive pain reducing drugs even though the effective dosage may hasten death	31	56	8	3	2	181

C. The Possibility of Medical Cure

	SA	A	U	D	SD	
1. The life of a dying patient should be prolonged, because a cure for his illness may be soon discovered	3	10	18	61	8	179

*The numbers listed in response categories are percentages.

SA = strongly agree
A = agree
U = undecided
D = disagree
SD = strongly disagree

signed waiver from the patient or responsible relative should be necessary for passive euthanasia of a patient expected to die shortly, although this is significantly less than the previous item. Apparently, a significant number do not feel that a signed waiver is necessary.

Eighty-three percent of nurses agree that "it is right for a physician to order pain and consciousness-removing drugs for a terminal patient, even though the drug may shorten life" (Table 6). Similarly, 87% feel that the patient should have the right to request and receive pain-reducing drugs which shorten life. Therefore, they tend to agree with what has been labeled the "law of double effect," which essentially means that they agree with the rationale of administering a pain-relieving drug even if such a practice may lead to the shortening of life. Though this procedure may be closer to the active termination of life, the nurses make a strong distinction in their attitudes between passive and active euthanasia. The distinction between the use of pain-killing drugs and the practice of active euthanasia seems to be based on the real intentions of the physician and the specific goals to be achieved with the use of the drug.

A main argument against the practice of euthanasia is that a premature termination of a patient's life may take place before the discovery of a *miracle cure* in time to save him. Surprisingly, the nurses, who emphasize the importance of medical cures, strongly indicate (69 percent compared to only 13 percent who believe in a new cure) they do not believe that, "the life of a dying patient should be prolonged, because a cure for his illness may be soon discovered" (see Table 6). Therefore, the nurses in the sample do not recognize the argument of a possible miracle cure as a valid reason for prolonging life.

The Influence of Religion

In the first statement in Table 7, Catholics and Protestants show similar attitudes on the maintenance of life-supporting instruments for patients, with adequate funds, on kidney dialysis. Considering statement two, Catholics are more opposed than Protestants to maintenance of life-sustaining treatment for the suffering terminal patient if the family so demands. On the surface, this item appears to contradict Catholic/Protestant differences commonly encountered throughout the study. However, Catholic nurses seem to react negatively to the suggestion that a family request be given paramount importance in deciding on the use of life-sustaining instruments. In contrast, statement three, which asserts that patients should have the right to receive passive euthanasia without fear of legal sanction, meets with significantly greater resistance by Catholics. The differential in Catholic/Protestant attitudes may well be pronounced because of the word "legal" as opposed to religious imperatives. The nurses of the two faiths were about equally divided on the less sensitive issue of the need for signed waivers for passive euthanasia of terminal patients (item 4). It appears that this final issue may not be as directly related to religious beliefs as are other topics.

Ordinarily, on a sensitive issue, such as active euthanasia (the taking of life through an act of commission, as opposed to an act of omission), a large difference in attitudes between the religions could be expected. The Catholic Church, however, considers "the law of double effects" to be acceptable. This means that the church approves of administering pain-killing drugs to suffering terminal patients in order to remove pain even though such treatment may indirectly hasten the patients' death.

Another factor which may also explain the lack of significant differences in the responses of Catholic and Protestant nurses is the possibility that the two groups are increasingly sensitized to the ideals of rapidly growing hospices and their commitment to giving high pain relief to the dying patient.

The belief in a miracle cure does not appear to be relevant to different perceptions by religion. Catholic and Protestant nurses share, to an almost equal degree, a lack of faith that a miracle cure may occur in time to save a terminal patient.

The Influence of Nursing Specialization

When considering a nurses's area of clinical practice, there is a common trend, clearly shown in Table 7. In all four items, geriatric nurses tend to be more opposed to the withdrawal of life-sustaining instruments. The trend approaches statistical significance when the

TABLE 7. Perspective on Clinical Issues Related to Terminal Illness by Religion and Medical Specialization

	Catholic						Protestant					
	SA	A	U	D	SD	N	SA	A	U	D	SD	N
Maintenance of Life-Sustaining Instruments												
1. Renal hemodialysis should be continued for patients with funds	14	19	16	37	14	51	7	26	20	33	14	117
2. Maintain treatment regardless of cost of family demands	4	42	32	22	0	50	5	48	23	19	5	121
3. Terminal patients should be free to receive passive euthanasia	27	57	14	0	2	51	37	52	3	6	2	120
4. A signed waiver of the patient or responsible relative should be needed for passive euthanasia	6	50	16	20	8	50	10	50	12	23	5	118
The Use of Pain-Killing Drugs												
1. It is right for a physician to order pain-killing drugs though they shorten life	25	57	10	6	2	51	23	60	10	5	2	120
2. Patients should be able to request pain-killing drugs though they shorten life	31	57	8	2	2	51	31	55	8	4	2	121
The Possibility of Medical Cure												
1. Wait for miracle cure	2	8	23	59	8	51	3	13	16	59	9	118

Degrees of freedom = 4

+ Values in X² columns are expressed as significance levels.
The numbers listed in response categories are percentages.

progressively greater gamma correlations in items one through four are examined.

Thus, statement one on the continuation of kidney dialysis meets with only slightly greater resistance from geriatric than nongeriatric nurses. The second statement, which suggests support for the family's request that life-sustaining treatment be continued, meets with

x^2+	Gamma	Geriatric						Non-geriatric						x^2+	Gamma
		SA	A	U	D	SD	N	SA	A	U	D	SD	N		
.554	.01	9	29	24	26	12	58	13	25	19	25	18	60	.730	.04
.398	.05	7	52	25	14	2	59	3	49	25	20	3	61	.776	.16
.037	.19	32	53	10	3	2	59	40	53	4	3	0	60	.464	.21
.852	.06	10	60	9	14	7	57	9	45	15	27	4	60	.278	.23
.995	.02	17	62	11	10	0	58	27	58	11	2	2	62	.175	.24
.969	.03	29	58	10	3	0	59	34	57	5	2	2	61	.608	.15
.720	.01	2	12	25	54	7	57	0	13	18	64	5	61	.672	.09

appreciably more resistance from geriatric than nongeriatric nurses. The issue of the patient's competence to make this request may precipitate the geriatric/nongeriatric differential. However, both medical specialty categories are in almost complete agreement about giving the patient this prerogative. Finally, the last item seems to give further confirmation that geriatric nurses have stronger convictions about the need to protect terminal patients from the abuses of euthanasia. Geriatric nurses have much stronger opinions about the need for a signed waiver prior to passive euthanasia.

In conclusion, geriatric nurses are more inclined toward maintenance of life-sustaining instruments. These nurses also show greater concern for the protection of the patient by placing progressively greater importance on the family's right to protect the patient, protecting the patient from his own inability to make the decision, and protecting the patient through the utilization of a signed waiver for permission to withdraw life-sustaining instruments. These attitudes of geriatric nurses may be the result of their greater involvement with dying patients.

Nurses in both clinical categories are highly approving of the use of pain-killing drugs even if they will shorten life, but geriatric nurses manifest noticeably less approval than do nongeriatric nurses.

Geriatric and nongeriatric nurses also share similar attitudes concerning the chances that a new cure might be discovered that would save the life of a dying patient. The chi square and gamma status show that there is no appreciable difference between the two categories. However, percentage differential does indicate that nongeriatric nurses have less faith in the possibility of a miracle cure.

SUMMARY AND CONCLUSION

The nurses make an obvious distinction between passive and active euthanasia. They find passive euthanasia highly acceptable and active euthanasia much less so.

The order of approval of the conditions acceptable for passive euthanasia reveals an orientation toward clinical and patient-centered conditions. Priority in permitting passive euthanasia is given to pain and personal suffering and secondary preference is given to the patient's personal reasons for desiring not to continue life in a demeaning manner. Psychological and financial hardships on the patient's family, as well as family or spiritual pressures, are ranked last.

Protestants and Catholics tend to find the conditions for passive euthanasia more acceptable than unacceptable. However, the percentage of Protestant "acceptable" responses always exceeds their Catholic counterpart for each condition.

The differential responses between the two religions are even more pronounced when referring to active euthanasia. Protestants accept active euthanasia more than Catholics do under all conditions. However, nurses from both faiths are generally substantially opposed to active euthanasia.

It was clear that geriatric nurses are significantly more opposed to passive euthanasia than nongeriatric nurses. However, nurses in both categories of specialization have strong feelings against active euthanasia. Geriatric nurses are more opposed to active euthanasia than are nongeriatric nurses, although the differences are not statistically significant.

The results illustrate that nurses do tend to see themselves as professionals, in their own right, capable of expressing disagreement with the opinions of the physician. For example, they do believe they have the right to request an inquiry by a medical board if they question the doctor's decision. In addition, nurses tend to concur that they can refuse to carry out a physician's legal order for euthanasia with which they disagree. However, they indicate greater readiness to carry out the physician's order for withholding medical treatment than to assist him in any clinical practice that could hasten death. In general, nurses in this sample feel they have the right to refuse to carry out a legal, professional duty if it conflicts with their personal values.

More than Protestant nurses, Catholic nurses believe they have the right to refuse to carry out the doctor's order. Perhaps they have become more sensitized to their rights since they have been confronted, more than the Protestant nurses, with the likelihood of having to carry out physicians' orders which may be contrary to their religious convictions. This may also explain why Catholic nurses have significantly stronger feelings about being just as qualified as physicians to make decisions in medical ethics. However, the Protestant nurses agree, to a significantly greater extent than Catholic nurses, that a nurse has the right to request an inquiry by a medical board if she believes a patient qualifies for voluntary euthanasia even if the attending physician does not.

Although religion was the most significant control variable in this study, it was not as strong an influence on the nurses' perspectives on clinical issues as might have been expected. This is probably because the attitudinal items do not sharply focus upon value differences in the two religions and/or the nurses' emphasis was placed more upon clinical imperatives than on ethical issues with respect to the use of life-supporting instruments or pain-killing drugs and the possibility of miracle cure. Thus, the two groups tend to have the same attitudes against the maintenance of life-sustaining instruments, except for one statement concerning the right of patients to request and receive euthanasia, which was significantly more unacceptable to Catholics. Also, the nurses of both faiths are about equally divided on the issue of the need for signed waivers for passive euthanasia of terminal patients. Similarly, nurses of both faiths approve, to an almost equal degree, the use of pain-killing drugs even if they may lead to shorter life. Catholic and Protestant nurses share a lack of faith that a miracle cure will be discovered in time to save a terminal patient.

Generally, the results for controls on medical speciality show distinct, though not statistically significant, trends. Geriatric nurses apppear to be more sympathetic to the suffering of the terminal patient and more opposed to the withdrawal of life-sustaining instruments. Geriatric nurses also indicated stronger feelings, compared to nongeriatric nurses, toward protecting the terminal patient. They displayed concern for the protection of the patient by placing greater importance on the family's right to protect the patient, protecting the patient from his own incompetency to make the decision, and the utilization of a signed waiver for permission to withdraw life-sustaining instruments.

Similarly, geriatric nurses exhibit distinctly less approval of the use of pain-killing drugs if they mean shorter life for the terminal patient.

From these findings, conclusions can be drawn that have some bearing on the test of the initial hypothesis. These conclusions can be stated in general terms as follows:

First, nurses distinguish clearly between passive and active euthanasia. Generally, they are in favor of passive euthanasia but they strongly oppose active euthanasia.

Second, nurses are patient-oriented when ranking the circumstances under which passive euthanasia could be used.

Third, religious (ethical) perspectives sharply divided nurses in response categories; Catholics registered greater opposition to all forms of euthanasia.

Furthermore, nurses appear to foresee a possibility for specific incongruencies between their roles and physicians' roles on matters related to euthanasia and the treatment of the terminally ill patients. This role incongruency may stem from a role distinction based on the differences between medical care, as provided by physicians, and health care, as provided by nurses (Wolinsky 1980). Such a distinction is made with reference to doctors' orientation toward cure and nurses' preoccupation with care (Kluge 1981). It may reflect the striving toward professionalism in nursing, particularly to achieve equal physician/nurse status within the medical institution. Medical ethics seem to provide nurses with an opportunity to assert independence and to build a coherent and distinctive nursing perspective.

The response of the nurses to this sample may have also been precipitated by what they see as a widespread callousness and insensitivity to ethical issues among physicians.

The findings clearly demonstrate that religious background has a clear impact on what nurses perceive to be an appropriate reaction to a doctor's directive that may not be compatible with their ethical values.

The most unexpected result of this study is the fact that religious background has little influence on the nurses' attitudes toward the maintenance of life-sustaining instruments, the use of pain-killing drugs and the possibility of a miracle cure (clinical issues). Regardless of religious background, the majority of nurses seem to hold the same attitudes toward these issues.

One possible reason for attitude convergence on clinical matters is that the Catholic church has come out openly for a medical practice of "no heroic efforts." The church has also accepted the administration of pain-killing drugs even if they may hasten the death of the dying patient (the law of double effects).

The data, however, unmistakably indicate that, because of their professional training, nurses accept certain clinical practices related to the treatment of terminal patients as imperative. Neither the Catholic/Protestant dichotomy nor the geriatric/nongeriatric distinction showed significant differences in the nurses' responses.

It is reasonable to suggest that nurses not only perceive of a measure of incongruency between their role and the physician's role, but also experience certain incongruency between ethical beliefs and clinical imperatives, especially when dealing with highly controversial and sensitive issues such as euthanasia and the proper treatment of the dying patient. This may force some nurses into situations where they experience "cognitive dissonance" between their religious ethical beliefs and their professional clinical training and practices. Such dissonance is apt to create role strains and role tensions within the health care team.

Finally, the limitations of this pilot study, particularly the low rate of questionnaire return, ought to be stressed. It should be made clear to the reader that these conclusions are suggestive rather than affirmative. Future research on the attitudes of nurses and of other professionals toward euthanasia and similarly controversial issues in the ethics of health care can benefit from posing more empirical rather than polemical questions. This research can also be advanced by utilizing theories of social psychological nexus between ethical values and clinical practices.

REFERENCES

Bates, B. (1972). "Nurse-physician dyad: Collegial or competitive?" In *Three Challenges to the Nursing Profession*. Kansas City: American Nurse's Association.

Brown, N. K., Bulger, R.J., Laws, H., and Thompson, D. J. (1970). "The preservation of life." *Journal of the American Medical Association, 211*(1), 76-81.

Carlton, W. (1980). "In our professional opinion." In *The Primacy of Clinical Judgment Over Moral Choice*. Indiana: University of Notre Dame Press.

Carney, T. P. (1979). *Instant Evolution: We'd Better Get Good at It*. Indiana: University of Notre Dame Press.

Crane, D. (1973). "Physicians' attitudes toward the treatment of critically ill patients." *BioScience, 23*(8), 471-474.

Downing, A. B. (Ed.). (1970). *Euthanasia and the Right to Death*. London: Peter Owen Limited.

Fletcher, G. P. (1970). "Prolonging life: Some legal considerations." In A.B. Downing (Ed.). *Euthanasia and the Right to Death*. London: Peter Owen Limited.

Fletcher, J. (1970). "The patient's right to die." In A. B. Downing (Ed.). *Euthanasia and the Right to Death*. London: Peter Owen Limited.

Flew, A. (1970). "The principle of euthanasia." In A. B. Downing (Ed.). *Euthanasia and the Right to Death*. London: Peter Owen Limited.

Freeman, H. E., Brim, Jr., O., and Williams, G. (1970). "New dimensions of dying.'' In G. Brim, Jr., H. E. Freeman, S. Levine, and N. A. Scotch (Eds.). *The Dying Patient*. New York: Russell Sage Foundation.

Friedson, E. (1971). *Profession of Medicine: A Study of the Sociology of Applied Knowledge*. New York: Dodd, Mead and Company.

Glaser, B. G. and Strauss, A. L. (1968). *Time for Dying*. Chicago: Aldine Publishing Company.

_____. (1965). Awareness of Dying. Chicago: Aldine Publishing Company.

Grisez, G. and Boyle, Jr., J. M. (1981). *Life and Death with Liberty and Justice: A Contribution to the Euthanasia Debate*. Indiana: University of Notre Dame Press.

Handin, D. (1973). *Death as Part of Life*. New York: W. W. Norton and Co., Inc.

Hogstel, M. (1977). ''Associate degree and baccalaureate graduates: Do they function differently?'' *American Journal of Nursing*, 77, 1598-1600.

Horan, D. J. and Mall, D. (1977). *Death, Dying and Euthanasia*. Washington, D. C.: University Publications of America, Inc.

Kluge, E. H. W. (1981). *The Ethics of Deliberate Death*. Port Washington, New York: Kennikat Press.

Levine, S. and Scotch, N. A. (1970). ''Dying as an emerging social problem.'' In G. Brim, Jr., H. E. Freeman, S. Levine, and N. A. Scotch (Eds.). *The Dying Patient*. 211-224. New York: Russell Sage Foundation.

Maguire, D. C. (1974). ''Death by chance, death by choice.'' *Atlantic Monthly*, *233*(3), 57-65.

Meyer, G. and Hoffman, M. (1964). ''Nurses' inner values and their behavior at work.'' *Nursing Research*, *13*, 244-249.

Meyers, D. W. (1970). *The Human Body and the Law: A Medical-legal Study*. Chicago: Aldine Publishing Company.

Nagi, M. H. et al. (1977-1978). ''Attitudes of Catholic and Protestant clergy on euthanasia.'' *Omega*, *8*(2), 153-164.

Nagi, M. H. et al. (1980). ''Euthanasia, the terminal patient and the physician's role.'' In *Education of the Medical Students in Thanatology*. New York: Arno Press/New York Times.

Nagi, M. H. and Lazerine, N. G. (1982). ''Death education and attitudes toward euthanasia and terminal illness.'' *Death Education*, *6*, 1-15.

Pellegrino, E. (1964). ''Ethical implications in changing practice. '' *American Journal of Nursing*, *64*, 110-112.

Popoff, D. (1975). ''What are your feelings about death and dying?'' (Part 1, 2 and 3) *Nursing*, *5*, 8-10.

Ramsey, P. (1970). *The Patient as a Person: Exploration in Medical Ethics*. New Haven: Yale University Press.

Reeder, J., and Haus, M. (1979). ''Nursing: Continuing change.'' In H. Freeman, S. Levine and L. G. Reeder (Eds.). *Handbook of Medical Sociology*, 3rd ed. Englewood Cliffs, N. J.: Prentice-Hall.

Schulman, S. (1972). ''Basic functional roles in nursing: Mother surrogate and healer." In E. Garley Jaco. *Patient, Physicians and Illness* 2nd ed. New York: Free Press.

Smoyak, S. (February 11, 1974). "Co-equal status for nurses and physicians." *American Medical News*.

Weisman, A. D. (1972). *On Dying and Denying: A Psychiatric Study of Terminality*. New York: Behavioral Publications, Inc.

Wolinsky, O. (1980). *The Sociology of Health, Principles, Professions, Issues*. Boston: Little, Brown and Company.

ADDITIONAL READING

Bahnke, J. A. and Bok, S. (Eds.). (1975). *The Dilemmas of Euthanasia*. New York: Dell.

Lasagna, L. (1968). *Life, Death, and the Doctor*. New York: Alfred A. Knopf.

Poslusny, E. et al. (1980). *Nursing and Thanatology*. New York: Arno Press.

Rabin, D. L. and Rabin, L. H. (1970). "Consequences of death for physicians, nurses and hospitals. " In G. Brim, Jr., H. E. Freeman, S. Levine, and N. A. Scotch (Eds.). *The Dying Patient* 171-190. New York: Russell Sage Foundation.

AFTERWORD

Grief:
Teaching the Hard Things

Florence E. Selder

"Sex! Drugs! Fear! Love! Grief! Rage! Conquest! What other business offers so much?" That is the lead-in for a poster about health care marketing in the 1990s. The promotional ad continues with the following: *"Breaking parity in the 1990s.* It will take more than advertising. More than physician bonding and product line development. The complex, the personal, the life-affecting emotions of your consumers must be tapped!"[1]

Marketing firms may be able to tap these complex and life-affecting emotions of health care consumers, but what about health care providers? Once these emotions are tapped, are professionals prepared to know how to deal with them?

For example, as a nurse goes off duty, a little boy who is dying with leukemia gives her an envelope and tells her to open the envelope the next morning. He gives his favorite doctor another envelope with the same instructions. He has two other envelopes: one for his brother and one for his parents. Tomorrow, when the nurse

---

1. Poster from McDonald Davis and Associates. (1988). Marketing/Communications. Milwaukee, Wisconsin.

129

opens the envelope, she finds five M & M's and a note. He writes that this is his will and thanks the nurse for taking care of him. The nurse gets teary-eyed as she experiences a sense of loss. Preparing and teaching about grief experiences such as these is both difficult and essential.

Grief is a subjective emotional state which a person may experience following a real or imagined loss. The loss is personally defined. The loss may be a death of someone, failure of one's health, losing employment, or giving up an addiction. The loss is the causal factor in a chain of response described as grief. People describe the response as physically uncomfortable, "I can't breathe, or I feel empty." The grief response is emotionally disorienting and may be described as, "I'm mad and then I'm sad, and I get so confused." The experience of grief is cognitively intrusive in that, "these thoughts won't go away." Since grief includes such a wide variety of responses, health practitioners require information about grief. In addition, practitioners need to know how to use this information in a meaningful way for themselves and their clients. To be effective, practitioners need to know how to deal with their own personal grief when it gets elicited by clients' grief. They also need to learn how to be comfortable with people who are grieving.

Why is it hard to teach about grief? It is posited that the things that are hard to teach are those things that are descriptive of our ordinary everyday realities. We create our realities in a manner that makes sense to us. These realities have a certain predictability about them. For instance, caring for clients recovering from an illness or surgery has a certain predictability about it. There is a certainty about performing procedures or administering therapeutics. These parameters of care giving are fairly well defined. On the other hand, care of a client who is grieving requires more than giving pills, doing treatments or teaching self-care. Fewer guidelines and less clinical information exists about the care of a grieving client. These clinical situations are also a lot less predictable. The client and the practitioner experience much more uncertainty. Their realities have been disrupted and this is not comfortable.

Why else is it hard to teach about grief? Teaching about the hard things triggers responses within ourselves and our students. As human beings, we have experienced many losses in the course of our lives and subsequently have grieved for those losses. There is the possibility that these losses, if unresolved, will be triggered by working with patients who are grieving. In these instances, there is a strong likelihood of personalizing the grief experience. In contrast, it may be easier to deal with a patient's diabetes if the disease is not part of one's personal, everyday experience.

Furthermore, our potential losses may be triggered. For instance, whenever I cared for a dying child who was the age of my son, I became more sensitive to his well-being. Uncovering the real, imagined, or potential grief may be uncomfortable. Teaching, learning, and speaking about it can recreate our earlier experiences and feelings.

Why else is it hard to teach about grief? It is hard to teach grief because of the complexity of the phenomenon. The teacher must be aware of the complexity of human beings and teach in a way that takes this complexity into account. Every student has emotional, physical, spiritual, cognitive and historical responses to phenomenon found in the health care situation. The student must be assisted in making distinctions for him/herself about these responses and how these may impact clients. For instance, it would be useful for a medical student to know his/her physical response to working with clients with grief. Does s/he stop breathing, or decrease his/her respirations, or distance from the client when the client is experiencing grief? Does the physical therapist give explanations of muscle groups to avoid an emotional discussion with the spinal cord-injured person who has begun to grieve over the loss of mobility?

The student must be able to explore his/her response to grief with the assistance of educators or more experienced clinicians. In the student's first client death, the student should explore with someone his/her feelings ("I felt helpless"), his/her thoughts ("I'm not prepared"), the physical sensation ("I feel heavy in my chest"), and historical data ("it reminded me of _____"), and the meaning ("Why does it happen to the young?"). Without an adequate exploration of the experience, the novice practitioner could use the discomfort s/he feels in the experience as a basis for unknowingly distancing from clients. This would be unfortunate for the practitioner and the clients.

Why is it hard to teach about grief? The things that are hard to teach are also hard to describe. There is no agreed language about grief. There are various stage theories about grief that attempt to describe this complex phenomenon. However, there is a great deal of variation in peoples' experience that is not easily captured by the word "grief." It may be useful to discuss grief in a variety of categories. For instance, students could categorize grief as "unsanctioned grief," such as losses occurring from alcoholism; "unrecognized grief," such as grief from loss of a pet or a job; "grey shadow grief" that is always there, such as from the death of a child; "intrusive grief," such as losses from a disease. The way grief is categorized doesn't matter. The categorization is only a way to have students begin to make distinctions and to begin to understand the great complexity of the phenomenon. Students can develop a language about grief that will serve them and share it with other students.

How to teach about grief? In teaching about grief, a teacher distinguishes between content and process. Content is the substance: the material or the units of information about grief a teacher selects to offer in a course or curriculum. The content of grief may be fixed in a generic course about death, dying, and bereavement. In some professional schools the concepts of grief may be integrated into an ethics course. In other schools, information about grief may be in sequence throughout the curriculum. At other times, content relevant to grief may not be formalized within a curriculum and it is assumed to be taught when a student needs it. The need is usually the first time a student is confronted with an experience, i.e., a dying person or death of a patient. Decisions of what, when and where grief should be taught will partially be made within the restrictions of the curriculum. These restrictions range all the way from those that are philosophical to content area discussions to time restrictions.

The second aspect of teaching is process. The process represents the context by which the student experiences the information that is being transmitted. This information may be emotionally charged and cannot be effectively delivered through lecture alone. Provision for students' responses to information presented should be made. The basis for ensuring that students have an opportunity to respond to the material is that inexperienced students will not easily utilize the information and transfer it to the clinical situation without reflection and discussion. The reflection ensures that inexperienced students are assisted in separating personal issues relative to grief from potential client issues. Use of a film as process may assist beginning students to identify their personal views, thoughts and feelings. Some students may have had personal experiences with loss, dying, and death in their family or other relationships. A process activity enables students to understand the complex phenomenon of loss and grief in the absence of clinical experiences. Additional activities may include writing one's own epitaph, writing a farewell letter, or creating clay or art products about a loss experience.

Films, planned activities, and small group discussions are means that can be used to elicit students' experiences with grief and their responses to loss. Teaching strategies that enable students to reflect on their grief in response to a loss will enable students to use their experience as a means of understanding clients' responses to losses relative to health and the illness state.

Teaching students information about grief and providing experiences to examine the information in a personal manner will assist future practitioners to do more than just tap the complex emotions of their clients; it will enable them to make a difference. Teaching about grief may be hard but it is also rewarding. As the nurse said about the boy who left her five M & M's, "I felt I made a difference."